# HOW
# JESUS
## HEALED THE SICK
## (and How You Can Too!)

---

Johannes Amritzer

Copyright © 2008 - Johannes Amritzer
All rights reserved. This book is protected under the copyright laws. This book may not be copied or reprinted for commercial gain or profit. The use of short quotations or occasional page copying for personal or group study is permitted and encouraged. Permission will be granted upon request. Unless otherwise identified, Scripture quotations are from the Holy Bible, New International Version®, Copyright © 1973, 1978, 1984 by International Bible Society. Used by permission of Zondervan Publishing House. All rights reserved. All emphasis within Scripture quotations is the author's own. Please note that Destiny Image Europe's publishing style capitalizes certain pronouns in Scripture that refer to the Father, Son, and Holy Spirit, and may differ from some Bible publishers' styles.

Take note that the name satan and related names are not capitalized. We choose not to acknowledge him, even to the point of violating grammatical rules.

DESTINY IMAGE™ EUROPE srl
Via Maiella, 1
66020 San Giovanni Teatino (Ch) - Italy

*"Changing the world, one book at a time."*

This book and all other Destiny Image™ Europe books are available at Christian bookstores and distributors worldwide.

To order products, or for any other correspondence:

DESTINY IMAGE™ EUROPE srl
Via Acquacorrente, 6
65123 - Pescara - Italy
Tel. +39 085 4716623 - Fax: +39 085 9431270
E-mail: info@eurodestinyimage.com

Or reach us on the Internet: **www.eurodestinyimage.com**

ISBN: 978-88-89127-62-9

*For Worldwide Distribution, Printed in the U.S.A.*

1 2 3 4 5 6 7 8/13 12 11 10 09 08

# Dedication

First of all, I would like to dedicate this book about healing of the body and soul to my loving Lord and Savior, Jesus Christ. Jesus, Messiah to the Jewish people and the hope for all people of every culture and ethnic group, is my greatest role model and best friend!

Imagine that the great and eternal God of this universe has revealed His deepest thoughts to humans in understandable terms in a collection of holy writings we call the Bible! Imagine that two thousand years ago, the great Creator of the universe, galaxies, solar systems, and small water molecules incarnated Himself as a sweaty carpenter from Nazareth in northern Israel!

Imagine that God in His love for you and me actually allowed Himself to be tortured and brutally executed on a Roman cross in Jerusalem, in order to completely identify with our sin. Imagine that He has risen from the dead, has conquered sin and evil, and is alive today! Imagine that it is possible to be completely forgiven from our sin, to receive healing for the body and soul, and to be restored through faith in Him!

Jesus, I am so fascinated by the example of Your life and Your great love! Your Spirit constantly intoxicates me. Yes, just the thought of what You have done for me chokes me up and brings tears to my eyes. You overwhelm me with Your love! You fill me with hope for the future, a surge of energy, and love for life! I love You more than life itself!

I would also like to dedicate this book to all of my coworkers at Evangelical Mission SOS International who are at the various bases and offices around the world. You are heroes in my eyes! All of you share the love of Jesus with me and my family as we live and work in daily discipleship-training and healing ministry. Maria and I love you as if you were our own children. All of Mission SOS's missionaries and workers, you are my true family members and closest allies!

I hope that this book will be an inspiration and cause an explosion of church growth through the healing power of Jesus! Your churches will grow and the good news will break forth into new ethnic groups when we boldly proclaim the Gospel of healing!

Finally, I would like to express a huge thank-you to all my brothers and sisters at our mission base in Smolyan, Bulgaria! I could not have chosen a more beautiful place to write this book than the heart of the kingdom of Pomacs, gloriously situated in the Rhodope Mountains, among bears, wild boars, and red deer!

Despite the total focus of your work, bringing salvation to the Pomac people, you took time to spoil me. I felt like the king of the Balkans for nine much-too-short days! Thank you for the salami and Austrian chocolate in the refrigerator and a huge, luxurious hotel room!

To Walter and Linda Zuniga, leaders of the Bulgarian base, you are my heroes and my greatest pride and joy! Thank you also to missionaries Annelie Persson, Lisa Hjertberg, and Marlene Segerstark for helping me with both the research and the compilation of this book!

For the sake of the unreached peoples,<br>
*Johannes Amritzer*<br>
Leader, Evangelical Mission SOS International

# Endorsements

Johannes is a real pioneer-evangelist, who goes out and seeks virgin ground everywhere. He finds it on the streets of Europe's dark cities as well as in remote countries like Lesotho or Burkina Faso, winning the lost for Jesus. His ministry includes prayer for the sick, and the miracles that follow authenticate his message. This book tells about it, and I highly recommend it.

*Reinhard Bonnke,* Evangelist
Founder of Christ for All Nations (CfaN)

I am so happy to be able to recommend to you this book and the overall ministry of Johannes Amritzer. If I could summarize Johannes' impact on my life, it is that he truly paints Jesus for me. When I hear him speak or read what he writes, I understand and feel the person and passion of Jesus a little more clearly than before. The pages of this book are filled with faith-building stories from both Scripture and present-day experience. The principles described here are more than just good theories. I can testify that I personally have seen them at work. In fact, I have become so addicted to seeing Jesus heal the broken that I have committed to attend and help sponsor at least one of Mission SOS's Signs and Wonders Festivals per year. As I have applied what is written in this book, I have seen God at work to heal the sick in my own ministry. I long for you to experience this as well. May you discover the living and miracle-working Jesus in your life as you read through this book.

*Jeff Leake,* Senior Pastor
Allison Park Church, PA
The LaunchPad Blog

Awe-inspiring, life-changing! You will be stunned and amazed as you read the real-life stories of people whose lives have been miraculously changed by the power of God. For Johannes Amritzer, healing and miracles are not just a book that is written but a lifestyle that is lived. I know you will be deeply amazed and challenged, as I have been, to believe God for greater works as you read these outstanding accounts. A must-read for everyone who loves Jesus!

*Ron Johnson,* Senior Pastor
Bethel Temple Church
Hampton, VA

# Table of Contents

|  | Foreword | 11 |
|---|---|---|
|  | Preface | 13 |
|  | Introduction | 17 |
| Chapter 1 | Healing in the Old Testament | 19 |
| Chapter 2 | Messianic Prophecies and the Twofold Redemption | 31 |
| Chapter 3 | Speaking Words of Healing | 43 |
| Chapter 4 | Faith in His Word | 49 |
| Chapter 5 | Drawing Near by Faith | 53 |
| Chapter 6 | Real Faith | 59 |
| Chapter 7 | Spirits of Sickness | 63 |

| | | |
|---|---|---|
| Chapter 8 | A Humble and Desperate Attitude | 67 |
| Chapter 9 | Prayer and Fasting | 71 |
| Chapter 10 | Be Specific | 75 |
| Chapter 11 | Always the Right Time | 79 |
| Chapter 12 | Shockingly Different | 83 |
| Chapter 13 | Gradual Healing | 87 |
| Chapter 14 | Demanded Attention | 89 |
| Chapter 15 | Address the Sickness by Name | 93 |
| Chapter 16 | Healing Through Confession of Sin | 97 |
| Chapter 17 | The Laying On of Hands | 103 |
| Chapter 18 | Acts of Faith | 105 |
| Chapter 19 | The Healing Touch | 109 |
| Chapter 20 | A New Thought | 113 |
| Chapter 21 | Clay on the Eyes | 115 |
| Chapter 22 | Healing of the Soul | 119 |
| Chapter 23 | Mass Miracles | 123 |
| Chapter 24 | Healing in the Book of Acts | 131 |
| Chapter 25 | Quotes From the Early Church Fathers About Healing | 141 |

| | |
|---|---|
| Epilogue | 149 |
| References | 151 |
| Healing Testimonies and Photographs | 153 |

# Foreword

THE END OF NOVEMBER 2006 WAS A historic time for all of us here. It was early Monday morning in the Rhodope Mountains when I knocked on the door of Room 208C at a hotel in central Smolyan. Johannes answered the door and exclaimed, "Hallelujah!" with a voice that has preached itself hoarse in more than 50 large festivals around the world and for the past 15 years has proclaimed the Gospel for thousands of people. His happy voice continued with a hearty laugh: "I'm so glad you are here! Now we are going to pray, Walter!" On the floor lay crumpled up paper, some Coca Cola bottles, and an empty Red Bull can; it appeared as though he had been writing well through the night. He looked at me with a smile and said enthusiastically, "Do you want to hear what I have written?!" "Of course," I said, and Johannes started to read aloud from the manuscript. His hoarse voice pierced through my heart, and tears ran down my cheeks as he read—it was very clear that the Holy Spirit's presence permeated the text.

This book contains more than 20 teachings on healing and many testimonies from SOS mission bases and festivals. Every page inspires health and faith. The author takes you directly into the festivals; and suddenly you are there, in the middle of a wave of signs, wonders, and miracles from Ethiopia, to the Philippines, to Ecuador, to a simple home in the Rhodope Mountains of Bulgaria. As I listened to chapter after chapter that November morning, my life was drawn even closer to my Lord Jesus and to His life of miracles.

I would like to thank my dear friend, Johannes Amritzer, for taking the time to visit us in Bulgaria and to write down healing miracles, experiences, and practical teaching from his everyday life. Mostly, I would like to thank our Lord Jesus Christ that this book has been written and that He continues to heal the sick.

At the beginning, we asked ourselves this question: Can one compile a book in just one week? The answer is yes, if one writes more than eight hours a day in hard discipline with the help of the Holy Spirit—and if your name is Johannes Amritzer.

*Walter Leonel Zuniga Mendoza*
Field Director of Mission SOS Balkan

# Preface

---

The book that you now hold in your hand is no official thesis on the subject of biblical healing. I make no claims as to theological depth or great intellectual capacity. This book was born on the battlefield and written on the road. The journey of discovery in the subject of biblical healing will continue for me, as an author, and hopefully also for you, as a reader, long after the epilogue has ended.

I want to continually learn more about miracle power in my relationship and walk with the Holy Spirit. I absolutely do not have all the answers concerning this. I am curious, open for enlightenment from the Holy Spirit, and longing for more practical experiences. The Bible, when studied in depth, is able to straighten out most of the questions, but I haven't received full clarity on the subject yet. Have patience with me, and maybe I will return in a few years with a better follow-up on the subject.

My prayer for this book is that it will be given and received as a practical guide for workers on the mission field's toughest front lines. This book was born and written during a Muslim rock-throwing in Ethiopia, during threat and persecution from security police in India, during an assault from a Bulgarian Mafia force on newly saved Christians on their way home from a sports stadium, and during a Jesus festival. In every one of these circumstances, the Word of God has enjoyed being confirmed, and the Spirit of Jesus has performed amazing miracles, signs, and wonders.

We have defiantly believed and preached to spiritually hungry people, and God has been faithful to His Word. This is no dry-and-dusty, untried theology but instead, what I have tested and experienced in sweaty, hard fieldwork during my first 15 years as an evangelist and missionary. I believe that this book is well suited for personal reading at home as well as group study. It is a handbook for missionaries and church pioneers to have in their start-up kit.

Healing is one of the most fantastic keys to Church growth and a breakthrough for new territory in the Kingdom of God among the unreached peoples. Healing opens the door to salvation for the Muslim, Hindu, and Buddhist who otherwise would never have allowed himself to be convinced that Jesus is the only way to God. When the blind see, the deaf hear, the tumors disappear, and the crutches are thrown into the air, then the masses will come running to repentance and salvation.

Believe me—I have tested, tried, and seen Jesus' healing power at work in approximately 50 Jesus festivals and countless conferences and cell groups up to now. This book contains many stories from my first years in ministry as well as from my recent experiences.

*Preface*

Disclaimer: All the testimonies I relate are retold from my memory, and therefore, all the details may not be 100 percent accurate. If someone who reads this book remembers an experience a little differently than I do, please forgive me. I have tried to retell the story as accurately as possible, but I have not researched all the details completely.

Introduction

# The Healing Ministry of Jesus

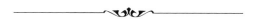

ALL DISCIPLES OF JESUS WANT TO BE LIKE Him and to do the things He did, right? Before we start to study Jesus' healing ministry in more detail, I would like to lay a foundation with a short study of healing in the Old Testament and the Messianic prophecies. This foundation comprises the first two chapters of this book.

After the first two chapters, we will begin to study how Jesus healed the sick according to the vivid and descriptive personal accounts in the Gospels. Jesus is our foremost example when it comes to practical healing ministry. In Chapters 3 through 22, we will look at Jesus' creative and unique way of treating the individual when He healed one or two sick people. I primarily portray the private and personal interaction between Jesus and the sick person, occasionally widening the circle to a small group of sick people.

It might be a little shocking when we discover that Jesus is not a psychotherapist or a scientifically schooled physician in His meeting and treatment of the sick. He is the Son of God, very straightforward and radical, and yet after His treatment, the sick are always made well and set free from what has ailed them.

Are Jesus' methods relevant in a modern and enlightened society with cancer research and state-of-the-art hospitals? The answer is yes, absolutely! Modern science and medicine are temporal; mankind can give medicines that only retard the progression of the disease but do not ultimately cure it. Jesus, on the other hand, with a gentle touch and word of comfort, intervenes and works a miracle that only He can do.

Let yourself be filled and smitten with the simple and uncomplicated faith that is found in Jesus Christ! In Chapter 23 we will do a short study of Jesus' ministry with the multitudes. Then in Chapter 24 we will run through the Book of Acts, ending in Chapter 25 with quotes from some of the early Church fathers to see what they have to say about healing. There is so much more that can be said and written on the subject of healing. I hope that this book will awaken your spiritual appetite and give you a hunger for more. Let's begin our trip through the Bible now!

CHAPTER 1

# Healing in the Old Testament

HEALING IS ONE OF THE MOST FANTASTIC KEYS to Church growth and breakthrough for new territory in the Kingdom of God. Healing opens the door to salvation for those who otherwise would never have allowed themselves to be convinced that Jesus is the only way to God. When the blind see, the deaf hear, tumors disappear, and crutches are thrown into the air, then the masses will come running to repentance and salvation.

Therefore, the book that you hold in your hand is not an official thesis on the subject of biblical healing. It is a practical manual for the reader to not only build a Biblical foundation for healing but also to be launched out in the power of the Holy Spirit to experience His power for healing today.

As you study the Word of God, your spirit will be awakened and your faith built. As you read about the real-life miracles that are taking place today, you will be motivated to action...to walk in the footsteps of Jesus...to see miracles of healing in your life and those around you.

The God that most of us have come to know through the New Testament story of a carpenter's son named Jesus is the same God that created the universe and the same God that revealed Himself to mankind through the people and history of Israel. In the Old Testament we see how God made a covenant (an eternal agreement or contract) with mankind. Through God's different covenant names we learn a little bit about His personality.

One of God's covenant names is *Jehovah Rapha*, which actually means "the Lord who heals" (see Exod. 15:26). The Hebrew word *rapha* also means "cure, (cause to) heal, physician, repair, thoroughly, make whole."[1] God has promised to bless and reward with complete health for body and soul everyone who follows the covenant.

With that thought in mind, join me on an exciting trip through the Old Testament stories. Allow yourself to be filled with an explosive faith in the God who healed the sick, raised the dead, and showed His power to mankind long before Jesus set foot on earth.

## Abraham and Sarah: Faith That Works Miracles!

*We Will Study Genesis Chapters 17–18 and 21*

Four thousand years ago the God of the Bible came down to earth. He made a quick visit to a small, dusty tent and showed himself to Abram. He promised Abram that he would become a father. He gave Abram the new name *Abraham*, which in Hebrew means "father of many nations," and entered into a covenant with him. Abraham was at this time quite advanced in years and physically *"as good as dead"* (Heb. 11:12). His wife's odds were not any better; Sarah was 90 years old and had gone through menopause (see Gen. 17:17 and Rom. 4:19). Over the years Abraham and Sarah had tried everything, but now they were beyond hope of ever becoming parents.

However, God promised Sarah that she would conceive and bear a son in exactly one year. When God finished speaking to Abraham, he knew that it would be exactly as God had said!

Abraham chose not to look at his own ability or circumstances, for they all pointed to the impossibility of the situation and spoke doubt and unbelief. Instead, Abraham decided to firmly believe in what God had said. He was *"fully persuaded that God had power to do what He had promised"* (Rom. 4:21).

Do you think that Abraham's neighbors thought he was overly confident when he suddenly started calling himself "the father of many nations," despite the fact that he was 100 years old and childless?! It is a miracle in and of itself that these two senior citizens, Abraham and Sarah, still made love to one another. The Bible says that Sarah *"became pregnant and bore a son to Abraham in his old age, at the very time God had promised him"* (Gen. 21:2).

How many Christians today have Abraham's unshakable faith in God's promises? How many dare say that they are healed after being prayed for in church, despite the fact that those next to them can see symptoms and proof that they are still actually sick? Do you think that we need more of Abraham's uninhibited and almost fanatical faith in God in the world today?

Abraham received a promise and had a covenant with God as a foundation for his faith.

How much greater then is the triumph of Jesus? His promises and covenant through His work of atonement is a foundation that is steadfast and immovable for our faith! (See Hebrews 8:6.)

Abraham dared to believe *"against all hope"* (Rom. 4:18a), when everyone, including his own wife, doubted and chose unbelief (see Gen. 18:12,15). How far does your faith reach?

Abraham dared to speak out his faith and call himself "father" long before Sarah's stomach even started to grow and stick out! Abraham's act of faith ultimately identified him as one of history's most famous fathers, and a forefather of God's own people, Israel! Try to catch hold of Abraham's miracle-working faith!

## Hannah: Walk in Faith, Act in Faith!
*We Will Study First Samuel Chapter 1*

Hannah lived in a country village, in the hills of Israel, during a time when most people had generally forgotten what God had promised to them. She lived together with her husband Elkanah and his second wife Peninnah, who had both sons and daughters. Despite the fact that Hannah was Elkanah's favorite wife, she was greatly grieved because she was barren; during those days people believed that a woman unable to bear children was worthless. However, Hannah was fortunate; she had a husband who deeply loved her.

Each year the family traveled to Shiloh, a nearby city, to offer sacrifices to God. During the trip, Peninnah would tease and provoke Hannah to tears. Most likely she was jealous that Elkanah loved Hannah more than he loved her, even though Hannah was unable to give him any children.

This year's journey was no different, and Peninnah started her ridicule of Hannah. Hannah, so distraught and overcome with grief, was unable to eat. When Elkanah saw Hannah's condition, he tried to comfort her. But Hannah knew the only thing that could bring her comfort was having a child of her own.

In her desperation, she went to the temple to pray and ask God for a child. She was crying so fervently that it echoed throughout the temple. She prayed so long and hard that her voice gave way, and finally only her lips were moving. The priest mistakenly thought that Hannah was drunk with wine and accused her, but she answered him, *"I was pouring out my soul to the Lord"* (1 Sam. 1:15b).

Hannah didn't have a gynecologist or a doctor to turn to. She didn't have a great amount of money to spend in a private clinic for infertility. She certainly didn't have any telephone numbers to adoption agencies in her desk at home either! Hannah went to the only doctor she knew of—and the only one who could help her: the Lord. After being in His "clinic," *"she went her way and ate something, and her face was no longer downcast"* (1 Sam. 1:18b).

The next day the family rose early and worshiped the Lord before they started the return trip home. Soon it was clear to the whole neighborhood that Hannah was with child!

Hannah knew that the Almighty God was the only one she could have turned to in a situation like this. She had mourned for so many years and felt that life was not worth living if she could not have children.

She cried out to God in her desperation, pouring out her heart and soul to Him, and prayed unyieldingly. She prayed through and gave birth to her miracle in faith!

When she had finished her prayer in the temple, she stopped feeling sorry for herself, wiped her tears, blew her nose, and strengthened herself again by eating some food. She acted in faith through prayer, and as a result, she received her request. Hannah's prayer of faith led her to mother one of the Bible's most important prophets, Samuel, which in Hebrew means "God hears"!

Meditate on Hannah's persistent and tenacious prayer and how she walked and acted in faith until she received her miracle!

There is no doubt that Jehovah Rapha, our heavenly doctor, has planned for us to have happy marriages blessed with lots of children! The covenant blessing we have with God includes the ability to conceive children: *"The fruit of your womb will be blessed"* (Deut. 28:4a) and *"The Lord will grant you abundant prosperity—in the fruit of your womb"* (Deut. 28:11a). These are just a few examples of a long list of blessings that God promises to His covenant people through Moses!

Read in Genesis 25:21 how Rebekah, though barren, conceived a child, or how God gave Rachel a long-awaited son in Genesis 30:22. Fill yourself with faith that God wants to fill the world with many happy mothers!

I would like to tell you briefly a wonderful story. In April 2004, Mission SOS together with Maranatha Mission (Trosgnistan) traveled to Migori in Southern Kenya to hold a campaign among the Luoa and Kuria people. During those few intense days, our Swedish team of 114 people prayed for many couples who were unable to conceive children.

One year later, my pastor and close friend Sven Bengtsson together with Curt Johansson, leader for Maranatha Mission (Trosgnistan), visited the same place to take part in a large pastors' seminar. They heard stories of how many infertile couples from Migori and surrounding areas had received prayer in the name of Jesus during our visit the previous year. The couples told with joy that finally they had become parents! Hallelujah!

## THE SHUNAMMITE WOMAN: NEVER GIVE UP!
*We Will Study Second Kings 4:8-37*

The woman from Shunem had everything a woman could wish for! She was rich, and after a prophetic word from Elisha, she miraculously received a child from God—the son whom she had always longed for.

One day, her little boy was out in the fields where the reapers were with his father. Suddenly he was afflicted with such a terrible headache that his father's servant had to carry him home. The boy sat on his mother's lap until noon, and then he died in his mother's arms.

Now the family was good friends with a well-known prophet, a holy man sent by God, whose name was Elisha.

Because Elisha would come and visit regularly, the Shunammite woman had fixed up a guest room for him to stay in. She carried the boy to Elisha's room and laid him on the bed. Believing that the God of Elisha could help, she hurried down the stairs to ask her husband to send her and one of their servants on a donkey to fetch Elisha. She would go herself and get the prophet!

Her husband didn't know that the boy had died and questioned her why she must leave in such haste. Her only response was that he should not worry, and that everything was all right.

The woman probably had a difficult time just trying to keep her seat on the donkey's back because she had instructed the servant not to stop or slow down, that they were to go as fast as possible until they reached the prophet.

When the prophet's servant Gehazi saw her from a distance, he ran to meet her and to see if everything was all right with her and her husband. She answered that everything was all right, but then made her way to Elisha and threw herself at his feet.

Elisha recognized her great distress as she told him why she had come, so he sent Gehazi with his staff to lay on the body of the little boy. However, the woman stubbornly insisted that the prophet Elisha come. Looking intently into his eyes, she said to him, *"As surely as the Lord lives and as you live, I will not leave you"* (2 Kings 4:30). So he got up and followed her home. She convinced the man of God to drop what he was doing and come to her aid!

When Elisha arrived at the woman's house, he went into the room where the boy was lying. When he saw that the boy was dead, he prayed and then laid himself over the body of the boy. He felt how the boy's body was getting warmer and warmer, so he once more stretched himself over the body of the boy. Suddenly the boy woke up, sneezed seven times, and then opened his eyes.

Elisha called for the woman and instructed her to take her son. When she came out of the room, she was carrying her son who was fully alive!

What can we learn from this story? The boy was dead, but the woman refused to accept it! She knew that his little heart had stopped beating, but she also knew that there was a man who carried the miracle power of God. She took a wild ride on a donkey and allowed nothing to stop her until she had arrived at the prophet's house. When she finally arrived, she dared to defy the word of the prophet and insisted that he come to her house to a boy who was already dead! She stubbornly held on to the only one she knew who had real contact with God, whereupon she got to see her son raised from the dead!

Have you ever thought that you didn't want to bother God with your requests and problems? Have you ever had a hard time believing in the power of God for your own life? Have you ever prayed, but then given up before you received the answer to that prayer?

Let yourself be struck with the contagious faith of the woman from Shunem. Be inspired by the kind of faith that is so stubborn and unshakable that it holds on until it receives the miracle from God. This woman's faith led to the complete restoration of her son's body!

How many people have you seen raised from the dead? I have not seen one yet, but I know I will...if I just decide to never give up!

In First Kings 17, Elijah, Elisha's spiritual father, met a poor widow whose son was sick and then died. He asked the woman to give the boy's body to him. Elijah prayed to God and *"the boy's life returned to him, and he lived"* (1 Kings 17:22). Read in Second Kings 13:21 how God revived a man back to life again just by being in the same grave as Elisha's bones. Even after Elisha's death and funeral procession, his body was full of healing and resurrection power.

*The Lord who heals* doesn't do miracles halfway, and His power in those of us who have chosen to believe and trust in Him is strong and mighty!

## Naaman: Swallow Your Pride!
*We Will Study Second Kings 5:1-5*

Naaman was the commander of the king of Aram's army, and he probably had a uniform decorated with lots of battle honors and medals. His reputation for being a brave and fearless soldier was well-known to all the men of that day, and everywhere he went he received respect and honor.

Nevertheless, Naaman was sick with leprosy, a sickness that gradually causes the flesh on the body to rot and fall off.

One day, a servant of Naaman's wife told her of a prophet in her homeland, Israel, who could heal the sick. So taking money and gifts, Naaman traveled to Israel to see this prophet.

In the meantime, a letter from the king of Aram reached Israel's king directing him to cure Naaman from his sickness. Tearing his robes, he cried out desperately, *"Am I God? Can I kill and bring back to life?"* (2 Kings 5:7). When the prophet Elisha heard of the king's dilemma, he sent a messenger to the king and said, *"Have the man come to me and he will know that there is a prophet in Israel"* (2 Kings 5:8).

Needless to say, Naaman's expectation was most likely high when he arrived by horse and chariot at Elisha's house. Surprisingly, Elisha sent out a message through his servant and instructed Naaman to go and wash himself seven times in the Jordan River.

The commander left angrily and yelled out:

*"I thought that he would surely come out to me and stand and call on the name of the Lord his God, wave his hand over the spot and cure me of my leprosy. Are not Abana and Pharpar, the rivers of Damascus, better than any of the waters of Israel? Couldn't I wash in them and be cleansed?" So he turned and went off in a rage* (2 Kings 5:11-12).

Then his servants came to him and said, *"If the prophet had told you to do some great thing, would you not have done it? How much more, then, when he tells you, 'Wash and be cleansed'!"* (2 Kings 5:13). Reluctantly, Naaman was persuaded to go down to the river and do what the prophet had told him. When Naaman came up out of the water, the God of Israel had done a complete miracle in his body! He was cleansed and free from his leprosy. Naaman cried out, *"Now I know that there is no God in all the world except in Israel"* (2 Kings 5:15b).

Naaman was a proud man and was used to getting things the way he wanted them. He had taken leave from his important job and traveled all the way to Israel to meet the prophet. But Elisha doesn't even come out to greet him. Then to add insult to injury, he is told to wash himself in a filthy Israeli river! The picture he had painted in his mind of how a healing should take place was totally destroyed. Naaman wanted to be healed, but he was angry when his healing didn't happen in the way or in the condition he thought it should.

The God of the Bible does not always come in the way that we think He should, nor is He packaged in the way we want. He always comes on His own terms!

Maybe you are one of those who have been sick for many years and still have not received your healing. You had been waiting for the great healing evangelist to come and lay his hands on you, but when he came, you didn't get well. Did you ever consider that maybe God was thinking of ministering his healing power through a girl who was working in the church café every Sunday, who had been longing to lay her hands on the sick?

God is not a respecter of persons. He sees to everyone whether they are of high or low rank. He wants to heal all who humbly bow before Him in faith. Humble yourself before Him, swallow your pride, and receive your miracle!

## KING HEZEKIAH: EXPECT A LONG LIFE!
*We Will Study Isaiah 38:1-5*

Among the kings of Judah there was no other king like Hezekiah. He was successful because he trusted and relied on God and did all that God commanded him to do (see 2 Kings 18:5-7).

In those days, Hezekiah became deathly ill. The prophet Isaiah came to the king and instructed him to put his house in order because he would not recover from his illness; he was going to die. When Isaiah left, the king turned his face to the wall and prayed. He was crying out to the Lord to remember him because he had done everything that God had asked him to do and had never let him down!

Then the word of the Lord came to Isaiah and told him to go back to the bedside of the king and say, *"I have heard your prayer and seen your tears; I will heal you....I will add fifteen years to your life"* (2 Kings 20:5-6).

After delivering the message, Isaiah instructed his servant to prepare a poultice of figs and apply it to the boils on the king's body. When the servant did this, Hezekiah immediately became well (see 2 Kings 20:7).

When King Hezekiah prayed to God, he received fifteen more years of life! God wants to give us a long life, and it is biblical to pray and ask God for it!

In Psalm 91:16, God says, *"With long life will I satisfy him,"* and in Proverbs, He says to remember His commandments and teaching, *"for they will prolong your life many years"* (Prov. 3:2). Solomon later writes to those who have received wisdom and says, *"Long life is in her right hand"* (Prov. 3:16a).

God's plan has always been to heal the sick and give long life to all people! There are so many more examples in the Old Testament. Miriam is healed from her leprosy in Numbers 12:10-15; King Ben-Hadad is healed from his sickness in Second Kings 8:7-14; and God heals a stream through his servant Elisha in Second Kings 2:19-22.

The more we study the Old Testament's stories, the more we are filled with faith in Jehovah Rapha, *the Lord who heals.*

So fill yourself with faith for a long, exciting, and adventurous life together with Jesus! Imagine that you hear the sound of your grandchildren's wild stories of all that God is doing through them! Or why not dream about being able to experience your grandchildren's children's laughter as they sit on your knee...?

The eternal God of the covenant, He who never breaks His promises but always keeps His Word, is the Lord your healer!

## Endnote

1. James Strong, *Strong's Exhaustive Concordance of the Bible* (Peabody, MA: Hendrickson Publishers), *Rapha* (#7495).

# Chapter 2

# Messianic Prophecies and the Twofold Redemption

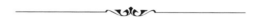

THE FALL OF MAN BROUGHT TERRIBLE consequences and curses, for both creation and mankind. Since that time, men, especially the Jewish people, have been waiting for a redeemer. They await someone who can establish harmony in creation and restore man to his original state of perfection.

The Creator of the universe often reveals secrets to His friends. In the Old Testament, there are prophetic pictures of what is to happen in the future. Sometimes these pictures are very clear and sometimes more obscure. The prophets, inspired by the Holy Spirit, describe the Messiah with astonishing detail and accuracy. One can sense the sweet aroma of Jesus in every Book. The Old Testament Scriptures are pulsating with salvation and healing. And so God's plan of salvation has been activated.

In year A.D. 30, just outside the city walls of Jerusalem, blood from a badly beaten back seeped its way into the wood grains of a cross. Jesus hung there with nails driven through His hands and feet. The spikes from the crown of thorns placed on his head penetrated deep into his scalp. The Messiah cried out with a voice that had been heard so many times in the streets of Jerusalem, *"It is finished"* (John 19:30). Then, before the eyes of everyone, He hung His head and died. The veil in the temple was torn from top to bottom, the earth shook, the mountains rumbled, and graves opened (see Matt. 27:50-52). Jerusalem's "scum of the earth" hung the God of the universe in the form of a man, along with a thief and a murderer. He had allowed Himself to be humiliated, abused, and killed so that He, once and for all, could redeem His creation: *"He Himself bore our sins in His body on the tree...; by His wounds you have been healed"* (1 Pet. 2:24). Then it was finished.

Your sins were completely forgiven and all sickness was completely healed in that very moment. No one will actually be healed *this* year—the whole of mankind *was* healed in year A.D. 30! That is why millions of people around the world will receive both physical healing and deliverance *this* year! Yes, thousands of evil spirits must loosen their grasp on people, because Jesus already delivered them on the cross two thousand years ago! It is finished! Shout it out! Believe it! Receive it! You can say, "I *am* saved, healed, and free," and the spiritual realities will rain down over your life!

## THE PASSOVER LAMB
*We Will Study Exodus Chapters 7–12*

Once again Moses walked through the corridors of the Egyptian palace. The sound of his staff hitting against the stone floor echoed with each step.

Several times before, Moses had come to Pharaoh appealing for the release of the children of Israel, who had been enslaved by Egypt for four hundred years. Each time that Pharaoh had refused to listen to Moses, plagues had come upon the land of Egypt. One time teems of frogs came up from the rivers and streams; at other times swarms of flies filled the air, grasshoppers ate up everything edible, hail rained down upon the livestock, and the Egyptians and their animals were smitten by boils. So now Pharaoh's court was wondering what his next threat would be.

Moses spoke the word of the Lord to Pharaoh. He warned him of the tenth and final plague that would strike if he didn't let the people of Israel go: *"Every firstborn son in Egypt will die"* (Exod. 11:5a).

Then Moses gathered all the children of Israel together and gave them instructions for the events of the next 24 hours.

Each family was to kill a lamb that was without defect. Then they were to take the blood of the lamb and wipe it on the top and sides of the doorframe. As it was getting dark, the families could be seen outside their homes with a butchering knife in their hands and blood on their clothes. According to Moses' instructions, they were to eat the whole lamb the same night. They were to eat with their clothes tucked into their belts, sandals on their feet, and a staff in their hands. They were to be prepared to leave their land of slavery when God delivered them.

That night a death angel went through all of Egypt and struck down every firstborn son, but it did not touch the homes of those who had the blood of the lamb on their doors.

The next morning Pharaoh released the children of Israel. He finally gave up, and the people were free to go.

Can you imagine an older woman, barely able to move, with a completely destroyed back? For the largest portion of her life, she had beaten bricks for Pharaoh's palace. Imagine also the man whose legs had been crushed under the huge stone blocks, who had not taken a step since the accident. And can you imagine the little girl who was born with a crooked leg?

While they were eating the Passover lamb, in faith, with their clothes tucked into their belts and staffs in their hands, God poured out a stream of healing power over the people.

The old woman was able to stretch out her body after a night's rest—and suddenly she noticed that she could now straighten her back! The man with the crushed legs looked with astonishment at two perfectly healthy legs! The little girl with the crooked leg was made completely well. During the night, as they ate the Passover lamb by candlelight, mass miracles took place as God healed the children of Israel! The Bible says, *"He brought out Israel, laden with silver and gold, and from among their tribes no one faltered"* (Ps. 105:37).

Here we see a clear Messianic prophecy. It is a foreshadowing from the Old Testament that points to reconciliation and gives us a greater understanding of what was accomplished on the cross.

The blood of the sacrificial Passover lamb saved the people from the angel of death. Eating the meat of the Passover lamb took away all their deformities, pain, and blindness and ultimately healed them from all their diseases. Similarly, Jesus, *"the Lamb of God"* (John 1:29), was sacrificed, and *"He entered the Most Holy Place once for all by His own blood, having obtained eternal redemption"* (Heb. 9:12). As the prophet Isaiah tells us, *"He was pierced for our transgressions…and by His wounds we are healed"* (Isa. 53:5).

The parallel is clear. Our Savior not only took our sin but also our sickness upon Himself. Jesus saved us from satan and the eternal death and also bought healing for our bodies.

For this reason, healing is already yours; the twofold redemption gave you a clean heart and perfect health for your body. We are completely healed today; it was accomplished two thousand years ago. Nothing needs to be added to the victory that the Lamb of God won on Golgotha. Then and there the curse of sin and death was broken, our salvation was secured, and our bodies were made whole. He has already done it! It is finished!

Now maybe you are thinking...if that is true, then why am I not healed? If everything is already done, why am I still in pain? Wait a minute now. Read the whole Book before you judge me.

## THE BRONZE SNAKE
*We Will Study Numbers 21:4-9*

The children of Israel, God's people, the apple of His eye, were free. And just like a teenager in love, God tried everything He could to take care of them and to charm them. He parted the Red Sea, served them manna and quail from Heaven, and from out of the rock, He gushed fresh running water.

Despite all that, the children of Israel started whining and complaining against God. It seemed as though they had forgotten the many years of slavery in Egypt. They forgot the tired and aching muscles. They forgot the stinging stripes on their backs from the daily whippings as they worked. Suddenly they remembered their poor and simple stews in Egypt as really good food.

Their sin of whining, complaining, and unbelief kept them wandering in the wilderness instead of entering the promised land. Furthermore, the children of Israel came out from under the covenant protection of God's hand, and they were attacked by sin's poisonous snakes.

Poisonous snakes literally entered Israel's camp and bit the children of Israel. Feverish, sweaty, and swollen from the poison in their blood, the people came to Moses full of regret and asked him to make an appeal to God.

Moses prayed, and God answered: *"Make a snake and put it up on a pole; anyone who is bitten can look at it and live"* (Num. 21:8). So for all who chose to look upon the bronze snake, there was healing and life.

When we read about the bronze snake, we see a clear Messianic prophecy; in fact, it is actually hard to miss the distinct parallel. Jesus Himself said in a conversation with Nicodemus, *"Just as Moses lifted up the snake in the desert, so the Son of Man must be lifted up"* (John 3:14).

Everyone hated the snakes; they were the cause of death. In spite of that, God commanded Moses to hang up a snake to bring healing to the people.

In the same way, Jesus, when He was crucified, identified Himself with our sin and suffering. When He carried His cross up to Golgotha, His beaten body was full of disgusting leprosy, depression, HIV, and all the different kinds of sickness and disease. Inside, Jesus carried all the sins of mankind—lies, jealousy, and dishonesty. He bore the sin of the whole world: *"God made Him who had no sin to be sin for us"* (2 Cor. 5:21).

The children of Israel only needed to look up at the snake hanging on the pole, and the poison of the snake immediately lost its power. In that moment, the people were made whole and free.

The same is true today. One look upon Jesus in faith brings freedom, forgiveness, joy, and…a body completely whole. Salvation and healing go hand in hand.

## The Groom

*We Will Study Song of Solomon*

I am so glad that the Song of Solomon is in the Bible! King Solomon's poetry is utterly boundless…the whole Book is full of love and romance. A bride sings the praises of her groom, and the groom brags about his bride. He compares her to gazelles, granite apples, doves, and herds of goats. But it's not just mushy romantic talk. It is a very strong prophetic illustration.

When you see the love between the bride and groom of the Song of Solomon, you understand the love that is to be present between Jesus and the Church, the Bride He is waiting for. *"They beat me, they bruised me; they took away my cloak..."* (Song of Sol. 5:7). In the Song of Solomon the bride was beaten; yet Jesus was also beaten for the Bride. He was beaten for His Bride's healing and salvation.

The bride spoke of her groom, *"Your name is like perfume poured out"* (Song of Sol. 1:3). The spoken name of Jesus is a healing balm poured out over your sores! Just the name *Jesus* breathes healing and can make one well.

I was preaching at a healing campaign in Karachi, Pakistan, in 1999. At the front of the platform, sitting in a wheelchair, was a woman with clubfeet whom I will never forget.

After listening to my preaching for about 15 minutes, she noticed, to her astonishment, that her deformed clubfeet had shrunk and were completely normal.

It was the power of the Word of God, Jesus Himself who created a faith within her that gave her a "go-get-it" attitude and produced her miracle.

Although she had not walked for many years, she jumped up out of her wheelchair, stumbled, and got up again. She pushed away everyone who tried to give her a helping hand, including her shell-shocked friends who couldn't even dare to believe that the impossible had suddenly become possible! She made her way up to the platform completely on her own! When she reached the top of the stairs, I saw her standing there with tears of joy streaming down her face. Spontaneously I started to dance around the stage, while the crowd cheered ecstatically!

It was the perfect conclusion to my sermon when people everywhere screamed out: "I am healed!" "I can see!" "I can hear!" "I can walk!" They understood that healing was ready and available to them! One by one they reached out, received by faith, and immediately started to tell each other what Jesus had done for them!

Everything is already done, but...it must be received in faith for healing to be manifested.

## The Suffering Servant
*We Will Study Isaiah 53*

At approximately the same time that Rome was founded and the first Olympic Games were held in Greece, a prophet, named Isaiah, emerged in the kingdom of Judah.

Isaiah was different because he refused to suck up to the government or try to be popular with the people. With raw simplicity and great integrity, he shouted out everything God told him to say.

I can picture him standing there with sweat breaking out on his brow and saliva spurting out of his mouth as he proclaimed the infallible word of God with a voice that was growing hoarse. Like a roaring evangelist, he preached salvation and repentance.

As the crowds gathered, he painted a picture of a man despised and rejected, beaten and tortured: *"He was led like a lamb to the slaughter,"* but *"surely He took up our infirmities....He was crushed for our iniquities...and by His wounds we are healed"* (Isa. 53:7;4-5). He continued to explain: *"Yet it was the Lord's will to crush Him and cause Him to suffer"* (Isa. 53:10a), *"and by His wounds we are healed"* (Isa. 53:7;5). Seven hundred years before it happened, Isaiah preached a crystal clear and detailed Gospel about Jesus. Did you notice that when Isaiah spoke about healing, he was suddenly speaking in the present tense: *"we are healed"*?

Talk about faith! Although Isaiah never saw Jesus physically, he saw Him spiritually. Seven hundred years before the birth of Jesus, Isaiah not only prophesied an unmistakable and detailed message about Jesus, but he also stood and boldly proclaimed healing through the wounds of Jesus! Talk about faith! The sacrifice had not yet taken place.

Indisputably what Isaiah prophesied in the Old Testament is confirmed in the Gospels of the New Testament. Today we can read the climax in the story of salvation. Receive your healing, you are healed!

Let us take a look at more prophecies of the Messiah found in the Old Testament. Ezekiel described "the Good Shepherd": *"I will search for the lost and bring back the strays. I will bind up the injured and strengthen the weak"* (Ezek. 34:16a). The Good Shepherd came to seek that which was lost and to bind up and heal that which was sick.

The purpose of the Son of God becoming incarnate man was not just to take us home to Heaven. The reconciliation includes all of your body, soul, and spirit. We are not to be hindered by any physical or psychological sickness.

It is much easier to preach if you have a voice that can be heard. It is significantly easier to push your way through a jungle to reach a people who have never heard the Gospel if you have a physical body that is working properly.

When the prophet Malachi prophesied, he described Jesus as "the sun of righteousness." Listen to these wonderful words: *"But for you who revere My name, the sun of righteousness will rise with healing in its wings"* (Mal. 4:2a). Can you see it? Righteousness will rise up for us, the sun of purity—Jesus—and healing follows directly after. Your physical healing follows salvation!

After four thousand years of darkness and pitch-black history, Jesus rose like a sunrise for mankind, and He brought healing with Him.

In February 2001, I visited the Turks in southern Bulgaria. One evening during the meetings, an uneasy, partially deaf Gypsy man showed up. Through a translator and sign language, we spoke of his 12- or 13-year-old son, who was with him. His son was also deaf and mute.

This father did not come for his own healing; he came for his son's. With tears running down his cheeks, he explained, "If only my son can be made well, our family will have a future."

This is my experience of the situation. I put my fingers in the boy's deaf ears. I prayed earnestly to God for a miracle. Then I put one of my fingers on his mute tongue and commanded the spirit of sickness to depart in the name of Jesus. Immediately the boy began to hear and tried to formulate some words. For us they were only incomprehensible sounds, but nevertheless it was clear proof that the boy's healing was reality.

More than two-and-a-half years later, I was back in Bulgaria. In the stairwell of a run-down apartment complex in one of the poorest Turkish and Gypsy quarters, I met a 15- or 16-year-old boy in a tuxedo and bow tie on his way to his own wedding.[1] With an exuberant shout, he stopped me as I was about to pass him. Through my Turkish friend and translator, he asked if I was "the holy man," the priest who had prayed for him almost three years prior so that he could hear and speak. I realized that it was the same boy who I had prayed for, and I was fascinated to tears that although a little slurred, his speech was now almost perfect, and he could hear everything I was saying!

"God is so good," said the young Gypsy bridegroom. "You have to understand, Johannes—my family and I had no future...but today I am going to marry a sweet young girl. It wasn't possible before, not even thinkable! But now I can work and earn my own money. Do you understand how happy I am that God sent you here? Now you will be my guest of honor at the wedding!"

Need I say more? My plans for that day were quickly changed, and I got to be part of a very different and exciting miracle wedding! What a celebration it was! God is great! God is so good!

## Endnote

1. In the southern European Gypsy culture, it is quite normal to marry early, around 15 to 16 years of age.

CHAPTER 3

# Speaking Words of Healing

*We Will Study Matthew 8:1-4*

AFTER HE PREACHED HIS FAMOUS "SERMON on the Mount," large crowds followed Jesus as He was making His way down the mountain into Galilee. Blocking the pathway in front of Him was a desperate man with leprosy who had pushed his way through the crowd. It was impossible to pass by him on the narrow little path that spiraled down the steep mountainside.

The man looked at Jesus straight in the eyes and said breathlessly, *"Lord, if You are willing, You can make me clean"* (Matt. 8:2b). Jesus saw that the man had a deep conviction for his healing. He saw the man's sincere, childlike faith, and I think that Jesus liked his style. This man wasn't beating around the bush with formal greetings or introductions—which might have been a good idea when talking face-to-face with a popular, miracle-working rabbi. Instead, he got right to the point and said what was most important.

Just as direct as the sick man's claim that He could heal, Jesus answered back with a quick and straightforward answer. Without doubt or hesitation, He said, *"I am willing. Be clean!"* (Matt. 8:3b). At the very moment He spoke, Jesus reached out and touched the man with His hand. Before the disciples had a chance to react over the "forbidden" action—touching someone with leprosy—the man received his miracle and was cleansed!

After hearing a faith-filled sermon by Jesus, this leper who had been condemned to an isolated life in quarantine had defied all the laws of the Jewish Torah and there on the hillside had received his long-awaited miracle. Jesus spoke words of creative healing power, and when He did, the disciples and all the others who were pushing along the path received a lesson in just how fast a healing can take place when instant faith comes in contact with Jesus' words of power!

The Gospel of John begins with Jesus being explained as the Word in creation: *"In the beginning was the Word, and the Word was with God, and the Word was God"* (John 1:1). It says that everything that was created was created through Jesus! *"Through Him all things were made; without Him nothing was made that has been made"* (John 1:3).

When God created the world, He simply spoke: *"And God said, 'Let there be light,' and there was light"* (Gen. 1:3). The Book of Hebrews says, *"By faith we understand that the universe was formed at God's command"* (Heb. 11:3a).

Jesus was the Word with a capital "W" that God spoke when He created everything we can see and touch: *"The Word became flesh and made His dwelling among us"* (John 1:14a). This means that when God was in the form of man, in the body of Jesus, on this earth, the world met *"all the fullness of the Deity liv[ing] in bodily form"* (Col. 2:9b). For this reason, it's not strange that when Jesus preached, the people said, *"What is this? A new teaching—and with authority!"* (Mark 1:27).

*Speaking Words of Healing*

When Jesus was awakened from His deep sleep in the middle of the storm on the Sea of Galilee, He rebuked the wind and waves and commanded, *"Quiet! Be still!"* (Mark 4:39), and immediately it became completely calm. The disciples became terrified and wondered: *"Who is this? Even the wind and the waves obey Him!"* (Mark 4:41).

Yes, Jesus was God—filled with the Spirit of God—but also 100 percent human. He was the perfect example for us. Jesus said, *"I tell you the truth, anyone who has faith in Me will do what I have been doing. He will do even greater things than these, because I am going to the Father"* (John 14:12).

If you are saved, the same Spirit is in you that was in Jesus! If you are baptized in the Holy Spirit, then you are wearing the same "working clothes" or fire that Jesus Himself wore here on earth! All you have to do is fill yourself with the Word of God and you will be able to speak words of power. These life-creating words spoken to the sick will immediately make them well.

So read the Bible a lot and meditate on the Word. God's Word will then flow out of your spirit through your mouth with words of health and strength to the sick. When you meet instant faith in people around you, speak the Word!

Proverbs puts it this way: *"The tongue has the power of life and death, and those who love it will eat its fruit"* (Prov. 18:21). Do like Jesus! Speak life! Create health!

In February 2001, Mission SOS held a festival in the city of Parzadjik in southern Bulgaria. Surrounded by a hungry audience of about 2,500 Turks and Roma, I suddenly heard the Spirit of Jesus say to me, "Bring forward all the deaf and those who are deaf in one ear!"

I had just finished my sermon and given an invitation, leading many in the prayer for salvation, but I immediately obeyed the Holy Spirit. Suddenly I received a vision where I saw Jesus and heard Him say to the deaf ears: "Be opened!" I described the vision for the people and watched the translators for the deaf sign out the message. When they understood, they eagerly nodded. Then, full of the Holy Spirit, I bellowed out:

"Deaf ears, be opened!"

After I lightly tapped eight of them who had come forward, those who were hearing impaired and some who were completely deaf suddenly received complete hearing! The excitement in the air was electric! The rejoicing and shouting knew no boundaries. I was stormed by a wild and miracle-hungry audience. I was blown away! When we didn't have the strength to pray for any more, my host and dear friend, Pastor Sasho Angelov, and I had to flee out the back door through a locker room.

Another time, an older lady in Sweden complained about her sore throat. "I can't eat or drink without excruciating pain," she said. "The doctors have noticed cell changes in my throat. Maybe it is the beginning stages of cancer?!" She was in a state of panic; fear was visible in her eyes. On the inside, I heard the Spirit of God say to me: "Say that she will be well in exactly three days." I repeated exactly what the Spirit had spoken, and the lady went to her home and I to mine.

Three days later she was standing by the window in her apartment; she couldn't sleep. She looked up to the stars and said in faith: "Now, Lord Jesus!" Suddenly it burned in her throat like a fire, and she was immediately healed! At her next examination, the doctors were unable to find even a trace of the cell changes in her body!

In the Indian state of Maharashtra, I stood on a platform in the city of Nagpur and proclaimed the Gospel to the Hindu masses. Suddenly I thought of the man I had seen in a vision the night before as I walked and prayed on the festival grounds. In my vision, he stood by a tree approximately 200 meters from the platform. He had a deaf ear but had received his healing through a "word of knowledge" (1 Cor. 12:8).

In the middle of my sermon, I shouted out into the crowd and pointed in the direction of the tree:

"Receive your healing now! Your left ear is now being opened!"

And there he stood, exactly as I had seen in my vision, and he received his healing. Hallelujah! I was almost as glad as he was when I listened to his testimony after the meeting.

I challenge you…do and be like Jesus! Speak words of healing!

CHAPTER 4

# Faith in His Word

*We Will Study Matthew 8:5-13*

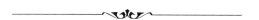

JESUS HAD HIS HOME AND MINISTRY base in the little fishing village of Capernaum, beautifully located on the northwestern beach of the Sea of Galilee.

Not far from Capernaum, on the western beach of the Sea of Galilee, was a large military colony—the Roman city called Tiberius. All of Israel was under Roman occupation.

One day Jesus was on his way home when a Roman centurion, most likely from Tiberius, came up to Him and asked for help.

You see, everyone had started talking about the Jewish "healer"—Jesus. Some of the Jews even thought that He was their long-awaited Messiah. So even this heathen officer believed...at least he believed in Jesus' ability to heal and that He had some connection with a great God.

The officer came to plead for help for his servant who was lying at home, paralyzed and in great pain. Jesus, straightforward as always, said to him, "Should I come all the way to your house and heal him...?" making no mention of the fact that He would defile Himself by going to visit the home of a heathen!

The officer quickly replied with words that surprised and impressed Jesus: *"Lord, I do not deserve to have You come under my roof. But just say the word, and my servant will be healed"* (Matt. 8:8). The officer had faith that if Jesus spoke the words of healing, the healing would be accomplished. As a centurion he understood that authority and submission to authority must exist in a well-working army. Just as his own soldiers obeyed their commanding officer, so sickness must obey the commands of Jesus if He were the Messiah!

The centurion showed great faith because he believed in the authority of both the physical and the spiritual world! Jesus exclaimed, "I tell you the truth, I have not found anyone in Israel with such great faith" (Matt. 8:10b). Wow! What a statement! This Roman officer's faith surpassed that of all the other Jews Jesus had met up until this point! To the officer, Jesus simply said, *"'Go! It will be done just as you believed it would.' And his servant was healed at that very hour"* (Matt. 8:13).

For healing to come to us, we need to learn to depend on Jesus and the Word of God! We must act on His Word! The Book of Proverbs emphasizes the importance of paying attention to the words of God, *"for they are life to those who find them and health to a man's whole body"* (Prov. 4:22).

We are to constantly have the Word before our eyes and kept within our hearts.

At the end of an outdoor meeting in the town square of Guayaquil, Ecuador, the Spirit of God said to my heart: "Do you dare to challenge them? In front of the people, bring a deaf person onto the platform and in My name open his ears. Demonstrate My power!" In obedience, I asked if there was someone completely deaf in the audience. Sure enough, there was, and they helped him up on the stage. There I stood in front of a very tense audience. Acting on the Word from the Spirit of Jesus, spoken to my spirit, I stuck my fingers in the ears of the deaf person and commanded them to be opened. Immediately he received his hearing, and complete chaos broke out when this Latin American audience understood that the power of Jesus was there.

Chaos is crowded, sweaty, and wonderful when everyone wants to be prayed for all at the same time.

Hallelujah! Have faith in His Word! I dared act in faith according to the inspiration and urging of the Holy Spirit, and a mighty miracle took place. Test it yourself, my dear friend! Boldness has its rewards!

CHAPTER 5

# Drawing Near by Faith

*We Will Study Mark 5:24-34*

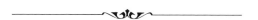

JESUS HAD BECOME QUITE A CELEBRITY in Galilee, and the crowds pressed in on Him as He made His way down the street. He was on His way to the home of Jairus, a synagogue ruler whose 12-year-old daughter was sick. Full of excitement at being in His presence, the crowds pushed and pressed in on Jesus. I don't know if celebrities wrote autographs during Jesus' day, but it is quite clear from this passage of Scripture that riot police and bodyguards didn't exist.

Maybe that was why no one saw or noticed her. She was not the type of woman one paid much attention to, and she brought no attention to herself either. She had never made her way out into public before. In fact, for the past 12 years she had been fighting a severe sickness of continuous hemorrhaging.

She had been to many doctors and had spent lots of money on different treatments, clinics, and cures. In truth, she had probably tried just about everything, including natural medicine and even some doubtful healing therapies. At any rate, she had spent all her money, including her savings, and yet her condition had continuously worsened.

So why was today so different? Because today was a now-or-never, win-or-lose day. For some time she had been hearing rumors of a miracle-working Jesus. And what had started in her heart as a little spark of hope had now grown into a full-blown conviction of healing. When she became an eyewitness to the countless miracles that took place during one of Jesus' healing meetings, all the doubt that she carried died. She began thinking to herself that if she could just touch the hem of His garment, she would be made well.

So there she stood, outside of Jesus' home in Capernaum, in the shade of sunset. With every miracle she witnessed, her faith grew. (See Mark 1:32-34.) *"Now faith is being sure of what we hope for and certain of what we do not see"* (Heb. 11:1).

Starting to speak to herself, she said, "There He is! I am going to go up to Him. All I need to do is touch the hem of His garment. There is such a crowd around Him...no one will even notice me."

And then she started to move. She fought her way through the masses. Not only was she weak and feeble in her body, but according to Jewish law, the bleeding classified her as unclean.

But then...finally! She took hold of the corner of Jesus' garment and let it go quickly again. *No one noticed anything,* she thought to herself, and she slipped back into the crowd. Immediately she knew: *I am well! I just know that I am completely healed!* All around her everyone was pushing and shoving, shouting and yelling; many were patting Jesus on the back, greeting Him and pulling on Him. Suddenly Jesus stopped, turned around, and said, *"Who touched My clothes?"* (Mark 5:30b).

As the people laughed, the disciples said to Jesus, *"You see the people crowding against You, and yet You can ask, 'Who touched Me?'"* (Mark 5:31). Come on! How could He ask such a question when so many were pressing in on Him and clinging to Him? However, Jesus continued to ask and look around; He wasn't deterred because He knew that He had felt power go out of Him (see Mark 5:30a).

The woman, trembling with fear, came and fell at His feet. Knowing what had happened to her, she told Him the whole truth. Jesus said, *"Daughter, your faith has healed you. Go in peace and be freed from your suffering"* (Mark 5:34).

What do we learn from Jesus here? We learn that there is a difference between how we draw near to Jesus and how we touch Him. Many people were touching Him, but there was only one person with the kind of faith that literally drew out power from the Son of God. Jesus detected—and always will be able to detect—a miracle-hungry person.

I have traveled to 55 countries and have met this kind of faith many times. In a great crowd of people who are cramming forward for prayer, I have felt the power and anointing increase so that it was almost "sucked" out of me. Someone took a hold of it and locked onto it during prayer, and I could feel how the physical power from Jesus pumped out through my arms and hands.

In the summer of 1992, a young Polish boy who was about 14 to 15 years old came to me for prayer. I will never forget what he said: "I want everything you have preached about!"

We started with a prayer of salvation and continued with a prayer to receive the baptism of the Holy Spirit and speaking in tongues. Next we went on to pray for healing from allergies, and then to deliverance from nicotine. Finally I started to prophecy over his future. After about 45 minutes of prayer, he said with an incredible, half-starved, passionate faith, "Is there anything more in the Bible that we can pray about?"

I felt completely exhausted and almost defeated when I answered him and said that I didn't know of anything more that we could pray about that night! I reassured him that I would be back the next day so he could come back if he had anything else to pray for. And he did. And we prayed and prayed.... His faith could almost wear out the most radical of faith preachers! I love the total lack of inhibition in new believers!

My dear mother-in-law, Siv-Britt, was also that kind of crazy, hungry Christian. At the end of August in 1999, much too early, she went home to be with Jesus. If you knew how much Maria and I miss her...the void that she left is very great sometimes. Oh, how I loved that woman! During my first few years as a new Christian, she was like a second mother to me. My upbringing had been rocky and unstable, and I really needed her.

I remember what a great impression she had on me as a newly saved Christian in 1990–91. Maria and I had just gotten together then Siv-Britt had become a Christian as an adult. She had tried most of what life had to offer with its pleasures, but now she wanted only to go to wild and radical Christian meetings. She wanted to sing worship songs, read Christian books, and listen to cassettes with faith teaching! There was nothing else that held any value for her. She was radical and wild, a real woman of prayer, a mighty "prayer warrior." She would fast for long periods of time and pray in tongues. She kicked off her shoes and danced in the aisles of the church and always went forward for prayer. She was truly a humble woman, and always wanted more. I remember one time when almost dejected, I took hold of her hand as she was making her way up for an invitation of salvation in a meeting and said, "You are definitely saved!"

She laughed when she saw that I was a little embarrassed for her and whispered back to me, "But at the next invitation I will go forward, just so you know…." What a wonderful attitude! Rather one too many times than not saved at all! Rather a little wildfire than no fire at all! The churches of this world need more Christians like Siv-Britt, that is for sure!

CHAPTER 6

# Real Faith

*We Will Study Matthew 9:27-31*

TWO BLIND MEN STUMBLED ALONG THE road leading to Capernaum. They had just heard that Jesus was passing by on His way home. Together they shouted out, *"Have mercy on us, Son of David!"* (Matt. 9:27).

It's interesting to note that Jesus waited until He entered His house to answer them. He actually let them follow, shouting after Him, all the way to His house! Most likely others were helping them, leading them, because it says that when Jesus came home, He went to them.

Then Jesus asked what one could consider a very strange question: *"Do you believe that I am able to do this?"* (Matt. 9:28). What a question! They had just followed Him all the way home, yelling as loudly as they could. They had even called him "Son of David," or in other words, "The Messiah." They acknowledged Him as the Redeemer whom the Jews were waiting for, and they desperately cried out to Him for a miracle.

Why did Jesus ask if they really believed that He could make them well? Wasn't their faith apparent to everyone? They were crying out so loudly that they were demanding His attention! Isn't it a little insulting to treat the sick and handicapped that way? Yes, if you just read this text on the surface, it could seem that way. However, Jesus actually asked a legitimate question.

Many times people who are sick just want to get a pat on the back. "Give me a little sympathy so that I have the strength to continue being sick." "Pray for me, Johannes!" "Feel sorry for me a little while, Johannes!"

Dear friend, I do sympathize with you. I would like to give you a huge, warm bear hug, too. I would gladly hold your hand and wipe the sweat off your brow when your pain becomes too unbearable to withstand. I could even sit by your sickbed for a whole night. I would gladly sit in a fishing boat and drink coffee with you for a whole day if you were in sorrow.

We dry many tears here at Mission SOS. But if you ask me to pray for your healing, then I am not so religiously sentimental. Empathy and compassion with the sick is very important. But when it comes to the prayer for healing, faith is even more important! That is why Jesus asked the question He did.

*"Do you believe that I am able to do this?"* Jesus asked. The blind men answered, *"Yes, Lord."* Jesus touched their eyes and said: *"According to your faith will it be done to you"* (Matt. 9:28-29). Immediately their eyes were opened.

With great joy and happiness they spread the news of what Jesus had done for them throughout the entire region. They left just as loudly as they had come. But now there was no longer a whine in their voice; rather, they made their way from the Master's house with rejoicing and extreme exhilaration.

During 2000, I was in the state of Uttar Pradesh, in the northern countryside of India. While there, I met a blind woman. With tears she told me her story through the translator. Six years prior she had started going to Christian meetings, and since that time she had been blind.

"The demons took my sight," she said.

"How?" I asked.

"Well," she said, "they warned and threatened me that if I didn't stop going to the Christian meetings that they would take my sight away from me. But in my entire life, I had never met such a warm atmosphere before. So despite the evil, demonic voices, I continued to go."

The Hindu woman wanted so much to be a Christian, but she couldn't get free from the grip of these demons. She didn't dare to believe that Jesus was really stronger than the evil spirits or that He was really for her.

I tormented her with the same question over and over again: "Do you really believe that Jesus can do this for you?"

She really didn't know for sure, but she still wanted me to pray for her.

The problem for me was this: I knew that she had received prayer so many times before without any noticeable difference or change to her eyes. Whether or not she or I believed anything would happen, I didn't want to be just another person in the long line of people who had religiously prayed for her. So I asked the question again: "Do you really believe?"

Since then, I have done this many, many times. I still ask the question, even at the risk of the sick person getting upset with me, which has sometimes happened. This one question is so important because prayer for healing cannot become a powerless, religious ritual.

As she cried, the demons started screaming out from her mouth. In the name of Jesus, I commanded the demons to give back the sight they had stolen from the woman. They answered much more wisely than I was able to pray. "We can steal," they said, "but only your Jesus can give sight to the blind." Sometimes the demons know more than a faith preacher and evangelist. Quickly I responded: "Thanks for reminding me."

Casting out the demons, I prayed for the woman's sight to be restored in the name of Jesus. Approximately one half hour later, she started to cry out from where she was sitting.

"I can see! I can see!" Suddenly she could differentiate colors and see everything plainly and clearly.

That is real faith!

CHAPTER 7

# Spirits of Sickness

*We Will Study Matthew 9:32-33*

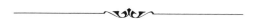

SOME PEOPLE MISTAKENLY BELIEVE THAT all sicknesses are caused by demons. It is true that there are sicknesses directly related to demon possession or demonic oppression. However, it is incorrect to suppose that that is the case for all sickness.

"How do you dare to claim something like that, Johannes?" Well, all the proof I need is in the fact that Jesus' healing ministry confirms this claim, and because Jesus Himself believed this!

It is important never to be too dogmatic. Instead we must learn to ask the Holy Spirit, our wonderful Helper, to reveal the source of the sickness before each specific healing that we want to see manifested.

Sickness has its root in Adam and Eve's fall, and there are definitely sicknesses caused by personal sin. At the same time, there are many who are sick without them actively or consciously sinning.

We live in a fallen world that is under a curse caused by man's rebellion. For that reason we all suffer to a certain extent from sin's ugly consequences. Sickness is one of those consequences. Therefore, sickness is not dependent on someone actively sinning. (We will come back to this subject of sin-related sicknesses and healing a little bit later in this chapter.) For now, let's look at some examples.

> *While they were going out, a man who was demon-possessed and could not talk was brought to Jesus. And when the demon was driven out, the man who had been mute spoke* (Matthew 9:32-33).

This story clearly shows us that there exist what we call "spirits of sickness." This man was mute because of demon possession, and after Jesus cast out the demon, the man began to talk. The sickness left with the demon.

Saul, the first king of Israel, appeared to be plagued with a spirit of sickness. When he started losing the kingdom to the advantage of the young man David, this spirit drove him into both violent rages and murderous conspiracies. First Samuel says that *"he raved in the midst of the house"* (1 Sam. 18:10, NASB). King Saul was driven by an evil spirit to the point of mental illness. Toward the end of his life, he was completely consumed with trying to keep his kingdom. He was neurotic, nervous, temperamental, jealous, and egocentric. The spirit that controlled Saul's life hated the simple, strong, childlike innocence of the clean spirit that was over the young servant and eventual commanding officer, David. This is no strange phenomenon for dictators and tyrants through the ages.

Personally, I believe that spirits can come, torment, and bind only that person who actively chooses to live in rebellion and sin. You can open the door for a spirit of sickness to have influence in your life. Then, through the confession of sin, the spirit is barred from access, and the door is closed.

When we choose to allow bitterness, jealousy, and control to rule and reign in our lives, we begin to live dangerously. We are opening up our lives for spirits of sickness. When we live in purity, we have nothing to fear. The evil spirits fear and flee from the person who is humbly submitted to God. *"Submit yourselves, then, to God. Resist the devil, and he will flee from you"* (James 4:7).

It is not unusual for people who have lived in immorality and lust to be delivered from a sexually transmitted disease at the same time that they pray for salvation. In the moment of salvation, when we confess our sins, many demons flee out of our lives.

It is also common that people are healed when they are baptized in water. The old house of demons is buried, and a new temple of the Holy Spirit is raised up from the baptismal.

Sometimes during the salvation prayer or while being baptized in water, addictions to nicotine, drugs, and alcohol disappear. When it doesn't happen at these times, it usually happens when the new disciple is baptized in the Holy Spirit and fire! Demons and demonic influence shun and avoid the fire of the Holy Spirit! I have seen demons of witchcraft leave screaming when we stand in the river right before the new Christian is to be baptized!

I'm sure many would like to criticize and dissect my teaching about deliverance from spirits of sickness, but I am not alone. Quite the contrary, I'm in good company. Jesus drove out the evil spirits and made the mute speak, although some said that it was the exorcism of demons: *"But the Pharisees said, 'It is by the prince of demons that He drives out demons'"* (Matt. 9:34).

Jesus is fantastic! Cry out to Him and confess your sins! He can deliver you from spirits of sickness!

We need to take one more example:

> *Then they brought Him a demon-possessed man who was blind and mute, and Jesus healed him, so that he could both talk and see* (Matthew 12:22).

During April 2006, Mission SOS was in the Ethiopian desert city of Harar. There was a Muslim woman from the Oromo tribe who was blind. At one of our festivals, she prayed the prayer of salvation. While she was praying, her eyes were opened, and immediately she started to see! The spirits of sickness fled, and salvation and healing came to this poor woman from the desert countryside! Many of her family and close relatives are believers and followers of Jesus today. Jesus is all-powerful!

CHAPTER 8

# A Humble and Desperate Attitude

*We Will Study Matthew 15:21-28*

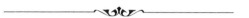

JESUS WITHDREW TO PRAY AND SPEND some time with His closest disciples and followers. Somewhere in Phoenicia (present-day Lebanon), outside the cities of Tyre and Sidon, Jesus tried to take a much-needed vacation. It is quite clear that Jesus wanted to hide from the constant stir and commotion around Him and His dynamic healing ministry. But the news had gone before Him; somehow it always got out to the public that the "celebrity" Jesus was in the area. So much for discretion and privacy!

Suddenly a woman from the area followed behind Him, screaming and crying out along the way, *"Lord, Son of David, have mercy on me! My daughter is suffering terribly from demon-possession"* (Matt. 15:22). The disciples, who were very tired, asked Jesus to send her away, *"for she keeps crying out after us"* (Matt. 15:23). The whole gang of Jesus' followers seemed quite bothered. Peter and John had just put on their "flip-flops" and were on their way with Jesus for a swim in the Mediterranean Sea. The whole timing of the incident breathed out "not now, wrong time!" Jesus said a little cryptically: *"I was sent only to the lost sheep of Israel"* (Matt. 15:24). When the woman finally threw herself at Jesus' feet and said, *"Lord, help me!"* (Matt. 15:25), Jesus answered with some very hard words. He said to a desperate mother begging for her daughter's deliverance from the occult, *"It is not right to take the children's bread and toss it to their dogs"* (Matt. 15:26). What Jesus said in His raw and rough way is actually freely interpreted as "Should I take miracle bread from the Jewish children and give it to a heathen dog like you?" (Note: This is Johannes' own interpretation, so blame him....) Ouch. Radical and hard! Why?

I think Jesus was testing the woman's attitude. How desperate was she? How much did she really want this miracle? What price was she willing to pay when it came to pride and prestige? Sometimes I wonder if pride and prestige isn't the currency that God wants us to use in exchange for something that otherwise is a completely free gift. Salvation and healing are gifts given to us by God on the cross through Jesus' blood and death, but unfortunately, these cannot always be received without "paying" a little bit in the form of stepping on our pride and dying to self (see Gal. 2:19b-20).

Now the woman answered in the most broken and humble way, saying, *"Yes, Lord, but even the dogs eat the crumbs that fall from their masters' table"* (Matt. 15:27). What an answer! What humble desperation! What a wonderful attitude! The woman essentially said: "Give me a crumb, Jesus! If I am a heathen dog, yes, that is possible, but I would like to take home just a few crumbs of your miracle bread to my daughter! Call me what you want, but I am so desperate that I have already died to myself." Jesus responded directly with these words: *"Woman, you have great faith! Your request is granted."* And as a result, *"her daughter was healed from that very hour"* (Matt. 15:28).

There are many who can tell how they received their miracles of healing when they finally surrendered their pride and prestige before God. Ask the leprous Assyrian commander-in-chief Naaman during the time of Elisha if you don't believe me. He didn't receive his healing until he obeyed the prophet of God and washed himself in the Jordan River seven times (see 2 Kings 5). Pride and prestige must die to benefit a humble desperation before God.

A non-Christian woman was about to have surgery after a hemorrhaging on the brain. The bleeding pressed on the brain right inside the skull bone. When she humbled herself, asked Jesus into her heart, and was on her way to be baptized in water, a miracle happened. We carried her down into the baptismal because she had such a difficult time moving one side of her body—a complication after the hemorrhage. She received the baptism of the Holy Spirit at the same time she was baptized in water. When we lifted her up out of the water, she was completely intoxicated with God's Spirit. We didn't know it then, but she actually had been healed at that very moment! There was no longer any need for an operation. The bleeding that had pressed so hard on her brain inside her skull was completely gone.

CHAPTER 9

# Prayer and Fasting

*We Will Study Matthew 9:14-29*

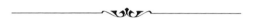

WE KNOW THAT JESUS FASTED 40 DAYS before He started His ministry after He was baptized in water and the Holy Spirit came upon Him (see Matt. 4:2). Long periods of prayer and fasting are wonderful; we need to learn how to practice praying with endurance and fasting a lot more, to follow Jesus' example, if we really want to have the same kind of miracle ministry that our Master had.

Jesus taught about the right way to fast in one of His most famous sermons: the "Sermon on the Mount" (see Matt. 6:16-18). He would never have taught His followers how to act and behave during a "right kind of fast," if He didn't take it for granted that they would also continue to practice it—i.e., to refrain from eating in connection with prayer. When Jesus was questioned about why His disciples didn't fast, while both the Pharisees and the disciples of John the Baptist fasted, He answered:

*"How can the guests of the bridegroom fast while he is with them?"* (Mark 2:19). Jesus continued, prophesying and promising that *"the time will come when the bridegroom will be taken from them, and on that day they will fast"* (Mark 2:20). In other words, Jesus expressly said that His disciples would fast. Sometimes Jesus needed to withdraw, pray, and possibly fast during a miracle campaign. Then we also need to do this.

On one occasion, Jesus returned from such a time of prayer together with His disciples Peter, James, and John (see Mark 9:1-8) to a large crowd of people. They were gathered around the remaining disciples, who were trying to drive out an evil spirit of sickness from a young boy. It didn't go so well, and the teachers of the law were arguing with the disciples, creating a lot of commotion. When Jesus arrived on the scene, things calmed down. Jesus was informed about the situation; He found out from the boy's father that he had come to the disciples for help, for the deliverance of his son. The father told Jesus about the attacks that the boy suffered, about how the demons would sometimes knock him to the ground. Sometimes the demons would seize him and make him foam at the mouth, gnash his teeth, and become stiff as a board. (See Mark 9:17-18.)

While they were talking together and discussing his diagnosis, the demons seized the boy, throwing him into convulsions and onto the ground again. The father became desperate and said that this had happened to him since he was a very little boy. The demon would throw him into fire or water and try to kill him. The father, who had seen the disciples' desperate attempt at trying to help the boy, did not doubt Jesus' ability to help. Jesus, however, gave him His usual little lesson in faith. The result was that the father exclaimed, *"I do believe; help me overcome my unbelief!"* (Mark 9:24). Jesus then commanded, *"You deaf and mute spirit, I command you, come out of him and never enter him again"* (Mark 9:25). The demon left the boy with a loud shriek;

he was finally free! Later, when the disciples were alone with Jesus, they asked, *"Why couldn't we drive it out?"* Jesus answered: *"This kind can come out only by prayer"* (some manuscripts say "prayer and fasting") (Mark 9:28-29).

Jesus taught here that there are certain demons that require prayer in order to be able to drive them out; and they may also require fasting in certain circumstances. Because this is about spirits of sickness, I will take the freedom to state that some sicknesses also need to be treated with prayer and fasting before healing can take place! Sometimes I hear questions like these: "You can't bargain with God in prayer, can you?" Or "If Jesus has already finished everything on the cross two thousand years ago, why do we have to fast and pray then?" Or "Does God really need my prayer and fasting in order to intervene and do a miracle?" No, one cannot bargain or manipulate God. Healing was already purchased for us on the cross two thousand years ago! It is finished! (See First Peter 2:24.) God does not need my fasting or prayers. His goodness and nature are eternal! (See James 1:17.)

Listen to me now! God does not need my prayer and fasting, but *I* need to fast and pray. *I* need to separate myself somewhere and be alone together with God in prayer. *I* need the discipline and order that a big fast creates in my life. Why? So that I can see clearly. Revelation gives birth to necessary faith. When I fast and pray for longer periods of time, I get a strong faith and a calm readiness for battle in my spirit. Demons hate Christians who fast because they are so disciplined. If you can say no to a spoiled stomach screaming for food, then you can say no to many other desires too. I need to fast and pray for my own sake. It creates the strong character that is absolutely necessary. Prayer and fasting make us holy, make us less spoiled and more thankful. Most of the strong breakthroughs in healing and deliverance from demonic oppression in Mission SOS have come at the end of a long period of fasting.

All glory to God! It is a fact that I cannot get around when I try to teach about healing. We in Mission SOS would not be able to do our pioneer work, church planting, and miracle festivals without a great amount of time with our loving God in prayer and periods of long fasting. We are completely dependent on God and daily miracles from Heaven in order to continue our work even for one week! We need to fast and pray more than ever!

CHAPTER 10

# Be Specific

*We Will Study Matthew 20:29-34*

JESUS WAS ON HIS WAY OUT OF THE OLD CITY of Jericho. As usual, crowds of people—pushing, shoving, and shouting—were following after Him. Two blind men were sitting by the side of the road when they realized that the miracle-working man called Jesus was about to pass them. The two men began shouting; it was impossible to shut them up. People told them several times to be quiet, but they shouted even louder. By now, Jesus had probably learned to live with this kind of commotion and the desperate cries for help from the sick and needy.

*"Lord, Son of David, have mercy on us!"* (Matt. 20:30). *"Jesus stopped and called them."* He was always teaching the disciples something new about healing, and this time was no different. Suddenly He asked the two blind men, *"What do you want Me to do for you?"* (Matt. 20:32).

One can wonder why Jesus asked them something so clearly obvious. I mean, wasn't it completely apparent to everyone that they wanted Him to give them back their sight? Well? Is it so obvious?! No. They may have had some other need, or they may have simply wanted to ask Jesus a question concerning the Messiah or the endtimes.

Sometimes I get angry when people see only Mr. Blind or Mrs. Paralyzed. Sick people don't *have* to have their entire identity wrapped up in their handicap. Even if sometimes it is that way, it doesn't always have to be. There are times people coming up for prayer say, "Just pray for me. God knows what it is." "Yes, of course...but why should *I* pray for you then?" I usually ask. Be specific! Specific and definite prayers receive specific and definite answers. I believe that Jesus asked them what they wanted Him to do for two reasons:

1. People who are sick are people who are suffering from a disease. They are not the sickness.
2. Jesus wanted them to be specific and definite in their request to Him.

Later in the passage, we read:

*"Lord," they answered, "we want our sight." Jesus had compassion on them and touched their eyes. Immediately they received their sight and followed Him* (Matthew 20:33-34).

Now, we know that it was healing they wanted that day, but we should not just take it for granted that the sick or handicapped always want healing when they request prayer.

I will never forget the woman, young yet withered away, in the electric wheelchair. After my sermon at a large meeting, she sat in front of me in the midst of all the others seeking prayer and help. Her friends pulled on my clothes, whispered, and asked me with tears in their eyes if I would pray for their friend in the wheelchair. When I came up to the woman, I felt hesitation in my spirit about praying for a physical healing because the Holy Spirit whispered clearly in my ear, "She is not baptized in the Holy Spirit." I said "Hello," and asked her name. Then after some short courtesy phrases, I asked her if it was possible that she was longing to be baptized in the Holy Spirit. She started to cry and answered that lately she had been longing for that. Then she added how moved she was by the fact that I didn't see her only as a handicapped person. "I thought you would be just like all the other preachers and pray for a physical healing. I am naturally thankful for that too, but it is really speaking in tongues that I am longing for, and I really need a stronger prayer life," she said. We prayed to Jesus, who baptizes in the Holy Spirit and fire, and she was filled with the Holy Spirit, bubbling and speaking in tongues for the first time in her life! She was so precious sitting there in her wheelchair with tears running down her face and fire from the Holy Spirit burning in her heart. Hallelujah!

CHAPTER 11

# Always the Right Time

*We Will Study Mark 3:1-6*

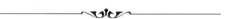

ON ONE OCCASION WHEN JESUS WAS visiting a synagogue, He met a man with a shriveled hand. Everyone was closely watching Jesus to see if He would heal the man on the Jewish Sabbath, a day of rest. The Jewish leaders, desperately looking for a way to accuse Jesus, considered that healing someone was "labor." For this reason, according to them, it was not appropriate for Jesus to heal the sick on the holy Sabbath, when no work should be done.

Jesus, with a combination of both anger and distress in His voice, asked the fault-finding, hard-hearted religious leaders, *"Which is lawful on the Sabbath: to do good or to do evil, to save life or to kill?"* (Mark 3:4). Then Jesus asked the man with the shriveled hand to stretch it out; when he did, he was made completely well at once. The Jewish religious and political leaders started immediately to conspire a plot to kill Jesus.

Here Jesus teaches that it is always the right time for a healing miracle!

What the prophet Isaiah said is really true: *"And by His wounds we are healed"* (Isa. 53:5b). Isaiah prophesied in present tense, speaking about something that would happen 700 years later as if it happened right then and there. When Jesus died on the cross, that is exactly what happened: By His wounds we were healed. Jesus healed us on the cross. When the disciple Peter talked about the same incident, he wrote in the past tense, as though it had already happened. What? Yes, look: *"By His wounds you have been healed"* (1 Pet. 2:24).

If it is done, it is done! We *have been healed!* That is why it is always the right time to proclaim and announce healing miracles, because it has already taken place! However, healing must be received in faith in order for it to be manifested.

Sometimes Christian people say to me, "I pray for the sick only when God tells me to do it. I want to act at the right time." They think that it sounds more spiritual if they say it that way. Some say, "I need to ask God if 'now' really is the right time for healing." How ridiculous! We don't need to ask God about what He has already said to us once and for all in His Word, the Bible! No, it even says in the Great Commission that *"they will place their hands on sick people, and they will get well"* (Mark 16:18b). That must still be valid, right?! Jesus said it! I want to be consistent and always pray for the sick, not waiting for special times and circumstances. It is always the right time to proclaim a miracle because it has already happened!

I was once invited to preach at a large Anglican stone church in Pakistan. This church form was very different for me, and the liturgy in the service bothered me so much that I lost all faith for the healing service they had asked me to come and give. I honestly thought that nothing miraculous could happen in this strange atmosphere of stone-faced people.

Out of pure stubbornness and the desire to aggravate a reaction, I gave an invitation to all those who actually would like to be saved and receive physical healing in their bodies. I asked them to come forward and gather around the altar. There was a complete explosion! There was a breakthrough with powerful miracles and several deliverances from demon possession. People were lying in piles all over the church, completely smitten with the power of God. A "half-crazy" homeless man who had gone around naked and dirty for many years was completely set free! It is always the right time for healing!

## CHAPTER 12

# Shockingly Different

*We Will Study Mark 7:32-37 and 8:22-25*

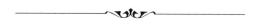

Up until this point, the disciples had seen and been part of most of the healing miracles. But on one occasion, Jesus did something shockingly different when healing a sick person, and they must have wondered what He was up to.

A multihandicapped man was brought to Jesus. The man was deaf and could hardly talk, and they begged Jesus to lay His hands on him. It says in the text that Jesus took him aside, away from the people, and put his finger in the deaf man's ears. So far so good, but then Jesus cleared His throat, spit, and touched the deaf man's tongue.

Maybe Jesus spit on His fingers and then put the saliva on the man's tongue; we don't really know for sure. But what we do know is that Jesus for some strange reason needed to spit, because it clearly says that *"He spit and touched the man's tongue"* (Mark 7:33b).

I am not going to try to find some deep, symbolic, charismatic, hidden explanation for this. Jesus spit. He needed to do it so that a miracle would take place. Why? I don't know. You may ask, "Why write about it then, if you don't know?!" That is exactly the point! I don't need to know and understand everything all the time; sometimes it is enough to obey and do what the Holy Spirit says to do, and miracles happen. It is a freeing thought, isn't it?

It says further that Jesus sighed and said, *"Be opened!"* (Mark 7:34). *"At this, the man's ears were opened, his tongue was loosened and he began to speak plainly"* (Mark 7:35). Though He loosened the tongue and opened the ears of this man, Jesus forbade those who were present there to tell where and how He had opened the ears and loosened the tongue. But they were not successful in keeping something so spectacular quiet, and we shouldn't judge them too hard for that! I don't think I would have been able to keep such an astounding and juicy healing miracle quiet either—I know that I would have at least told my wife!

But then...He did it again! Next they brought a blind man to Jesus and asked Him to lay His hands on the man. (See Mark 8:22.) It sounds almost religiously pompous to tell Jesus what to do: "Lay your hands on him." Jesus did it His own way.

Maybe that is exactly why I love Jesus so much, because He was never predictable and never exercised worn-out religious methods and formats. He did not come up with "seven keys to your healing miracle" or an "ABC of solutions." The way He went about spitting in people's faces, especially those of sick people, Jesus probably would not have gotten many speaking engagements in churches and conferences today!

In the city of Bethsaida, in Galilee, Jesus took a blind man by the hand and led him outside of the village. Wonder why?! It says: *"When He had spit on the man's eyes and put His hands on him, Jesus asked, 'Do you see anything?'"* (Mark 8:23b). Jesus spit on his eyes. Jesus spit on his eyes. I will write this even a third time just to aggravate you, so enjoy it: Jesus spit on his eyes.

"Why, Johannes?" You and I need a spitting Jesus. The world needs a spitting Jesus! Why are there no paintings with this motif? Why are there no icons or church ornaments of the spitting Messiah? Why do they sell oil and water in cute little bottles in Israel and not the saliva from some old saint? Ask the next time you are in a souvenir shop on a trip to Israel: "Do you have any healing saliva in a bottle or jar?"

I want to purposely provoke you. It has become so pompously religious in Christianity today that Jesus hardly has a chance to do His miracles! We need to change that! We need to break the bonds of "fine-culture Christianity" and slaughter a few "holy cows"!

CHAPTER 13

# Gradual Healing

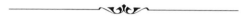

WHAT MORE CAN WE LEARN FROM THE spitting Jesus? Well, that sometimes healing can come to us gradually, by successively getting better and better.

We read about the blind man in whose eyes Jesus spit: *"He looked up and said, 'I see people; they look like trees walking around.' Once more Jesus put His hands on the man's eyes. Then his eyes were opened, his sight was restored, and he saw everything clearly"* (Mark 8:24-25).

We need to learn to not give up but to continue to pray again and again. Every time we pray we are closer to a complete healing. Sometimes healing comes immediately, sometimes gradually, step by step.

I prayed for a woman in Bulgaria in April 2002; she was paralyzed from her waist down. She had sat in a wheelchair for many years. Her leg muscles were withered; her legs looked like cooked spaghetti that just hung in the air when we lifted her up out of the wheelchair. We prayed for her several days in a row and finally she walked! She didn't walk the first day we prayed, but she did get back some of the feeling in her legs. Then she received the ability to move and balance, which improved little by little for every day that went by...until on the fourth evening of the festival, she walked, using her wheelchair as a kind of walker. I was so happy for her. I don't know why it is that way sometimes, and I have no opinions on it either, but I think that it is just as wonderful when someone is gradually healed as when it happens immediately.

Another time I saw a woman rise up out of her wheelchair and start walking in the middle of my message. The God of the Bible is good! Keep holding on, you who are still longing to receive your miracle. We will pray again. It will get better and better every time—only better and better, my dear friend.

CHAPTER 14

# Demanded Attention

*We Will Study Mark 10:46-52*

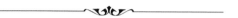

When Jesus left Jericho with His disciples, a large crowd followed after them. By the side of the road sat a blind beggar named Bartimaeus.

When I am home at bedtime, my children, Alicia and Adam, love to hear me tell this story before they say their prayers and I kiss them goodnight. We usually call it "Bible theater," in the Amritzers' kitchen. This means that Daddy tells the story and simultaneously plays all the characters and roles. Sometimes Mommy makes an impressive acting effort, but of course in much smaller roles. But anyway...

When Bartimaeus heard that it was Jesus from Nazareth who was on His way by, he started to yell and shout at the top of his lungs.

No one could stop him. There were many who tried to quiet him and spoke sternly to him, but he just yelled and shouted more and more loudly for each reprimand and warning he received.

If you are desperate for a miracle—and in this case, the opportunity seemed to be right for a healing to take place—why not give it all you've got?! Just go for it! Demand attention! What do you have to lose?

Jesus stopped on the way and said, *"Call him"* (Mark 10:49). *"Cheer up! On your feet! He's calling you"* (Mark 10:49), the people said to the blind man. Bartimaeus threw his cloak aside, jumped to his feet, and came to Jesus. *"What do you want Me to do for you?' Jesus asked him. The blind man said, 'Rabbi, I want to see'"* (Mark 10:51).

I love this part of the story, the actual point of contact between the blind man and Jesus. True, Bartimaeus demanded Jesus' attention, but now when he is standing close to Jesus, he says humbly, almost whispering: "Rabbi," meaning "teacher" or "master," "please make it so I can see again." He was now in front of Jesus. He stood so close that he could almost feel and hear Jesus' breath. He didn't need to scream any longer. So Jesus said, *"Go, your faith has healed you"* (Mark 10:52).

How did the blind man respond? As soon as he received his sight, he began to follow Jesus (see Mark 10:52). Bartimaeus followed Jesus. Maria, Alicia, Adam, and I are also following Jesus along His road. Jesus has actually done miracles for all four of us!

I think back to a festival series that Maria, I, and the Mission SOS team sponsored in cooperation with another Swedish missions organization. The festival was held in Pakistan during the winter and spring of 1999. We visited three large cities and held healing meetings and pastor seminars, in Karachi, Lahore, and Islamabad. We had just finished the last festival meeting in Karachi where many had demonstrated and testified about their miracle experiences from the platform. Lines of people were still circling down the stairs to the outdoor stage where they would tell about the wonderful ways Jesus had delivered them that night.

It is a wonderful and sweaty chaos that just has to be experienced to be understood. It is like a wonderful poison, a heavenly drug that you get addicted to and need more of once you have tasted it. There is nothing quite so fantastic as a large healing festival!

The audience at this particular festival in the city of Karachi I will never ever forget as long as I live. With help of soldiers and security guards, we were to flee into the waiting cars behind the platform that took us to our hotel, when something happened.

During the following few minutes, a scene played out that is forever etched on my memory. People stormed forward screaming and shouting, trying to reach us, but were withheld by the security guards. When we were finally sitting in the cars and our chauffeurs were trying to drive out from the festival area, desperate, miracle-hungry people threw themselves against the windows of the cars. They held up their sick children and pointed to the lifeless bodies they were holding in their arms.

It was the shouting, the tears, and the desperation of these needy people that made our hearts break, as though they had been torn up into small pieces. We had prayed and ministered to people for hours already and were completely wiped out, but there was no end to the need. The masses continued to come in a steady stream for us to lay our hands on them and pray. Yes, I wanted to stay and continue to pray all night, but the security guards could guarantee our safety for only a little while longer, so we had to go to the hotel....

I have seen similar scenes many times after that campaign in Pakistan in 1999. I have experienced the same desperation in different countries, sometimes among my beloved unreached Muslims, Hindus, or tribal people. They have stolen my heart—or more rightly said, stuck a knife right through it—with their desperate hunger for Jesus and His miracle-working power. Their style, when they demand attention, always makes me very humble and reflective. I have such respect for the sick and the relatives assisting them, pressing themselves forward in the crowd, never giving up their faith for a miracle.

CHAPTER 15

# Address the Sickness by Name

*We Will Study Luke 4:38-39*

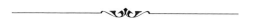

*Jesus left the synagogue and went to the home of Simon. Now Simon's mother-in-law was suffering from a high fever, and they asked Jesus to help her. So He bent over her and rebuked the fever, and it left her. She got up at once and began to wait on them* (Luke 4:38-39).

WHEN JESUS HEALED SIMON PETER'S mother-in-law, He spoke to the fever in command form. Jesus treated the fever as if it were a personality that was attacking the woman. Jesus clearly addressed the sickness by name and commanded the fever to leave, and it left.

Sickness is never a blessing in disguise from God, as some people wrongly believe. Sickness was not part of God's plan and purpose for us when He created us. Sickness is always an attack on a person's life, even if the sickness is congenital.

Congenital sickness is not only an attack on an individual but also against a whole family.

Sickness is always a curse—ask the person who is sick and has great pain if it is not exactly what one would call suffering or a curse. If you think that I am too healthy to claim this, then ask my father or my father-in-law, who both have been battling cancer for several years now. Listen to what they have to say.

Just because Jesus spoke to the fever as if to a personality and in some cases drove out spirits of sickness, it doesn't mean that all sicknesses are demonic personalities. The Bible does not say that Jesus rebuked a spirit of fever, but that He spoke sternly to the fever. Peter's mother-in-law was not possessed of an evil spirit of sickness, but she was attacked with a sickness. She would not have been bedridden if she were not under attack; she was plagued with attacks of fever. You might say, "Explain now, because I don't understand! What is the difference?"

When we live in this world, we are attacked and tempted with all sorts of things (see James 1:13-16). Sometimes we sin. If I get angry or say something bad, I don't automatically become possessed with a "demon of anger," but without a doubt I have given in to an evil influence or an evil persuasion. The solution is not to cast out the demon of anger but to ask for forgiveness and draw near to God instead.

We can be attacked with sickness like this also, and the solution is not exorcism but rather a prayer for healing in faith, where we speak to the evil and it has to yield. Start to speak to sicknesses as personalities and you will see that your authority increases and that you pray with greater conviction and weight. Evil must yield to the name of Jesus!

The apostle Paul said about Jesus: *"Therefore God exalted Him to the highest place and gave Him the name that is above every name, that at the name of Jesus every knee should bow, in heaven and on earth and under the earth, and every tongue confess that Jesus Christ is Lord, to the glory of God the Father"* (Phil. 2:9-11). Jesus is the name above all names! Use it! Colds, rheumatism, allergies, AIDS, syphilis, polio, and hepatitis are all names of sicknesses, right? But the apostle Paul says that Jesus' name is above all names, which means that Jesus is above all names of sickness, and they all must bow their knee and confess that Jesus is Lord!

Can you see AIDS and herpes lying on their knees reluctantly—but nevertheless loudly and clearly—confessing that Jesus has won a glorious victory on the cross and that His name is greater and stronger than theirs?

Jesus said this of His name: *"Until now you have not asked for anything in My name. Ask and you will receive, and your joy will be complete"* (John 16:24). The apostles Peter and John had just healed a lame man so that he was running and jumping, when Peter said: *"By faith in the name of Jesus, this man whom you see and know was made strong. It is Jesus' name and the faith that comes through Him that has given this complete healing to him, as you can all see"* (Acts 3:16).

I will never forget the wild healing service, the one I shared with you in Chapter 15, when this truth came down like a bomb of revelation in my spirit. The Holy Spirit whispered, "Speak to the sicknesses as persons." The sicknesses became the enemy, and I spoke sternly to them in the name of Jesus. What a difference it made immediately! Many visually handicapped people received perfect sight when I called out, "Stigmatism be gone, go!" Many deaf ears opened when I suddenly started to speak to "Mr. Deafness," and said that I was tired of him and told him to take a hike!

CHAPTER 16

# Healing Through Confession of Sin

*We Will Study Luke 5:17-26*

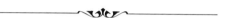

"AND THE POWER OF THE LORD WAS PRESENT *for Him to heal the sick*" (Luke 5:17b). The power to heal was clear and apparent for everyone, and Jesus was, as usual, surrounded by both people who supported Him and the hostile, fault-finding opponents. The religious elite, the Jewish leaders of that time, were constantly examining Jesus. They were weighing, bending, and twisting every word He said in order to find a way to entrap Him.

It was extremely crowded in the house where Jesus was teaching and healing the sick. His disciples as well as the Pharisees and teachers of the law were all there. Four men came carrying a paralyzed man on a stretcher. Because of the great crowd, they were not even able to come into the house. So they climbed up onto the roof and started taking the shingles off; they lowered the lame man down right in front of

Jesus, right there where He was teaching. At the very least, this was ferocious and very aggressive faith, but Jesus seemed to like the situation and said to the man on the stretcher, *"Friend, your sins are forgiven"* (Luke 5:20). A great gasp went through the crowd because Jesus dared do something so radical as forgive sins. Thoughts were spinning, and there was a buzz throughout the whispering crowd in the completely packed house.

The scribes thought, *Who does He think He is, that Jesus? What a blasphemer! It is only God Himself who can give forgiveness of sins!* Some of them probably wondered why Jesus spoke about forgiveness of sins to the paralyzed man: *It isn't forgiveness he needs most; it's healing.* Jesus, who knew what the people were thinking in their hearts and minds, asked a rhetorical question to His slightly shaken crowd: *Which is easier: to say, 'Your sins are forgiven,' or to say, 'Get up and walk'?* (Luke 5:23).

It was so quiet you could hear a pin drop; a strange mixture of tenseness, slight criticism, and almost shocked surprise hung over everyone who was gathered in the crowd. *What is He going to do?!* Suddenly, Jesus said these very loaded words: *"But that you may know that the Son of Man has authority on earth to forgive sins... I tell you, get up, take your mat and go home"* (Luke 5:24).

Jesus proved His authority with the miracle that He performed, teaching us two very important truths:

1. Jesus forgives sins, and forgiveness is actually more important than a physical miracle. (It's better to go to Heaven limping than to go to hell healed.)

2. Sometimes healing and the forgiveness of sins are connected to one another, and in order for a miracle to take place, sins must first be forgiven through confession before God.

Jesus not only saw the faith of the paralyzed man and his half-crazy friends, but He also saw that the sick man sought after the forgiveness of sins.

When the lame man and Jesus' eyes met, Jesus satisfied the most important need in him. It was primarily his sinful soul that sought forgiveness and redemption. When the man knew that he had been forgiven, he could receive a miracle without delay: *"Immediately he stood up in front of them, took what he had been lying on and went home praising God"* (Luke 5:25). He went home primarily forgiven, but also completely healed in his body. What a wonderful day!

I have already said earlier that sickness is not always because of sin in a person's life. At the same time, in this book, I do not want to steer away from the fact that there are sick people who actually are ill because they have opened up the door in their lives to an attacking and evil devil, through active personal sin. If you can become ill because you have sinned, then you can only get well through confession and the forgiveness of sin.

The Bible supports these radical claims very clearly. When the apostle Paul taught on how to be and to act before partaking of communion, he spoke primarily about the importance of examining ourselves (see 1 Cor. 11:28). Paul said: *"For anyone who eats and drinks without recognizing the body of the Lord eats and drinks judgment on himself"* (1 Cor. 11:29).

Paul meant that by taking communion lightly, without seriously confessing our sin or regularly examining ourselves, it could actually be dangerous for us physically. A lax attitude toward things concerning holiness can cause grave consequences for us, leading both to sickness and a shorter life.

In the first letter written to Corinth, Paul said very clearly that lack of self-insight and sound self-examination had created the weak health condition and state of the church in

Corinth at the time of his letter: *"That is why many among you are weak and sick, and a number of you have fallen asleep. But if we judged ourselves, we would not come under judgment"* (1 Cor. 11:30-31).

One of Jesus' half brothers, James, puts it this way in his letter: *"Therefore confess your sins to each other and pray for each other so that you may be healed. The prayer of a righteous man is powerful and effective"* (James 5:16). James encourages us to confess our sins and then pray for each other, and he says that confession can be the actual criteria for a miracle: so that you may be healed.

One time in Sweden, I prayed for a woman who was 65 years old. She was suffering from a terrible joint disease—rheumatism. When I prayed for her, I clearly saw in my spirit that the disease was like a huge tree growing inside of her. The tree had its roots all the way down to her feet and out through her toes, and the branches made their way up into her arms and out through her fingers. The Holy Spirit, whom we always and in every situation must learn to ask for advice, said to my spirit: "A root of bitterness that was once planted as a small seed has grown up into a large tree." I told the vision to the lady, and she started to cry and tell her life's story.

She and her husband were saved early on in life, when she was around 20 years old. About the same time, she was baptized in the Holy Spirit and started speaking in tongues. At age 25, she was rejected and abandoned by her husband for another woman. She was left alone to fend for herself and take care of their three small children. Because of this divorce 40 years ago, a root of bitterness had been sown in her heart, and it grew and grew through the years until it was a huge tree. She was very unhappy, very sick, and in much pain on a daily basis.

We started by praying together and confessing the bitterness as sin. It didn't matter that she had been treated badly by her former husband, because now what was most important was her life and freedom, and not his. Then, while we were praying and confessing, she started to pray in tongues. Suddenly she opened her eyes and said, "I haven't spoken in tongues since the divorce 40 years ago!" She continued to happily praise the Lord and babble in tongues.

"I believe you are going to be healed now too," I said.

"Yes! I can feel it in my whole body," she shouted loudly.

Two days later she came back beaming all over and told of the long walks without any pain or problems at all in her body. Hallelujah!

Let me point out for the reader that the only way to be able to tell the difference between what is what, to learn to discern, to be able to separate apples and oranges, is through prayer in the Holy Spirit. You must learn to ask the Holy Spirit for help and advice. He wants to help you and give you the necessary discerning spirit in your meeting with different kinds of people and sicknesses. Jesus never performs a miracle exactly the same way twice, and every healing is unique in its own wonderful way!

All sickness and all suffering have their roots in the sinful fall of man, when the curse affected all mankind: *"Therefore, just as sin entered the world through one man, and death through sin, and in this way death came to all men..."* (Rom. 5:12). Sickness is thus always a result of someone's sin (maybe Adam's sin), but not always because the one who is sick has sinned.

An innocent child of a young prostitute in the slums of Kampala is born with HIV. The child suffers from the disease and awaits an early death, because of someone else's sin. Sometimes a child is born with a deformity, because the mother took drugs during the sensitive pregnancy or was abused by an abusive boyfriend or mate. A whole village gets sick because they all drink the same poisoned water, and many are suffering from being exposed to radioactive rays from a nuclear power plant accident. We can definitely become victims of sickness as long as we live in this world, even if we try to walk in the light (see 1 John 1:7a) and live a clean life. If you have confessed your sins, then you should naturally not live in fear; instead, we should stand together in faith for your miracle.

I wear glasses and have fought against nearsightedness my whole life. I try to walk before God with a clean conscience and have never felt condemned because I have bad eyesight. But at the same time, I realize that I at times am too comfortable to even seek a healing when I can live so well with glasses on. I also have a part of my identity in my glasses, and they have almost become a part of my adult personality. It is, of course, not good that one can learn to live with the fact of needing glasses as normality, and that is exactly why I nowadays seek healing for my eyesight and constantly build up my faith. One day I will receive the healing that Jesus won for me—it actually belongs to me! It will come! While I stand in faith for my coming eyesight-miracle, I preach and continue through life with joy over everything that Jesus has done!

Worship and sing in your wheelchair! Preach Jesus with a walking stick for the blind in your hand! Nothing can stop a dangerously positive Christian on his way to healing!

CHAPTER 17

# The Laying On of Hands

*We Will Study Luke 13:10-17*

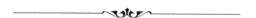

IN A SYNAGOGUE, JESUS MET A WOMAN who had been crippled by a spirit for 18 years. When Jesus saw her, He called out, *"Woman, you are set free from your infirmity"* (Luke 13:12b). Then He laid His hands on her, and she immediately straightened up and was healed! A wonderful deliverance from yet another spirit of sickness and a physical healing had taken place! (See Luke 13:16.)

Jesus practiced what we call, in our Christian religious terms, "the laying on of hands." The problem with the laying on of hands in many Christian circles today is that it has gotten a little blown out of proportion as the specific way of mediating healing.

In Christian cultures and countries, Christians hardly understand anymore what a powerful practice the laying on of hands actually is. There is nothing wrong with the practice itself; instead we have to blame a powerless, dead, and ritualistic Christian religiosity as the culprit. The laying on of hands must regain its original status and the high expectation that it deserves.

I believe that one should be careful in practicing the laying on of hands as the only prevalent healing method, something that has unfortunately become quite common. When the Holy Spirit leads us to lay our hands on someone, a transference of power occurs. This is really one of the most powerful ways to impart healing and deliverance to someone. Our arms become like electric power lines and our hands just as dangerous for sickness as electric outlets are for small children. In you resides God's power plant, and your hands become like hot irons that burn away all sickness. The Bible says that during Paul's visit to Ephesus, *"God did extraordinary miracles through Paul* [a fantastic missionary and adventurer]" (Acts 19:11). Everything that came in contact with him or *"touched him"* (Acts 19:12) became full of God's healing power, and people were immediately healed.

Jesus, our great example, says to His disciples after His resurrection and right before His ascension: *"They will place their hands on sick people, and they will get well"* (Mark 16:18b). What a promise from Jesus! There is not even a hint of doubt when Jesus confirms that this is how it is going to be! It just is!

CHAPTER 18

# Acts of Faith

*We Will Study Luke 17:11-19*

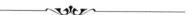

As usual, Jesus was out on the streets. He was always on His way to new and exciting destinations and healing miracles in His contact with the different kinds of people He met. On His way into a village in Samaria, He met ten seriously ill men from a leper colony. They lived in seclusion, quarantined outside of the villages and cities in specially designated places according to the health laws of that day.

From a distance, they shouted out to Jesus, *"Jesus, Master, have pity on us!"* (Luke 17:13). Jesus answered, *"Go, show yourselves to the priests"* (Luke 17:14). Why would they go and show themselves to the priests?

Well, we could compare it to present-day doctor examinations. The priests made a diagnosis after examination, and they declared someone clean or unclean, sick or healthy. In the case of leprosy, they could even order quarantine, given the extremely contagious nature of the disease. You did not go to the doctor or priest for a reexamination if you had already received a diagnosis, unless you believed yourself to have become better or completely well.

These ten men who were very ill with an ugly disease called leprosy were doomed to isolation from their healthy relatives and friends for the rest of their lives. But Jesus said, "Go and show yourselves to the priests!" *But we are sick,* they probably thought, *and one does not show himself to the priest until he is completely well!* It could seem a little contradictory, but it was an admonishment for them to "go in faith," as if they had already become well.

> *And without faith it is impossible to please God, because anyone who comes to Him must believe that He exists and that He rewards those who earnestly seek Him* (Hebrew 11:6).

According to the laws for leprosy in the Jewish Torah (Law), one would facilitate the priest's examination by making a few preparations. The Book of Leviticus requests that before they come to the priest, those who are to be "cleansed" shave off all the hair on their body, bathe, and put on newly washed clothes. Jesus radically challenged these ten men, who were still sick, to do all of this: "Go and show yourselves to the priests!"

Yeah, but, you might ask, weren't they Samaritans? One of them was, the passage tells us (see Luke 17:16). Because Samaria was specifically named, I assume that the others were Jews, or at least most of them were. They probably followed the Torah's instructions before going and having themselves examined. Talk about acting in faith!

They didn't just immediately go to the priests after their encounter with Jesus, like one can be led to believe when reading this lightly. No, they shaved and bathed their sick bodies, and then they put on clean clothes and started their journey together to show themselves to the priests. They did all of this in faith from what Jesus had said for them to do. On the way to the priests, they walked straight into the healing power of Jesus. All ten men became well when they acted in faith upon what Jesus had requested that they do, but only one returned to say thank you. It was the Samaritan.

Jesus responded to the Samaritan in a way very characteristic of Himself: *"Were not all ten cleansed? Where are the other nine? Was no one found to return and give praise to God except this foreigner?...Rise and go; your faith has made you well"* (Luke 17:17-19).

Yes, Jesus is quite direct, and I never cease to be fascinated by what an evident faith He had. Jesus already seemed to know that all ten men were healed. The only thing He was surprised over was that not all of them came back to give thanks to God. And so the whole story ended with these words: *"Your faith has made you well."*

Yes, faith is so very important. Actions done because of faith in the promises of God will usually release miracles. Co-operation with God becomes so clear in acts of faith: *"Therefore I tell you, whatever you ask for in prayer, believe that you have received it, and it will be yours"* (Mark 11:24).

In other words, Jesus' kind of faith is about believing before you have even received an answer to prayer. You must believe that you have already received what you have prayed for and expect it before it has become a physical reality.

This is precisely what happens all the time at our "Signs and Wonders" festivals in Mission SOS. People from all different kinds of cultures, but primarily Muslim and Hindu people, respond even while we are still preaching the Gospel. They "come and get it" in wild, unrestrained, and almost aggressive faith—faith in the miracle power of Jesus!

In November 1997, on the island of Luzon in the Philippines, I was preaching the Gospel to some tribes in the jungle.

An older man from a former head-hunting tribe ran up to the platform every evening on every altar call and got everything before anyone else could. I didn't even have a chance to finish the invitation for salvation before he was already up at the front. I didn't even get to finish my teaching on the baptism of the Holy Spirit before he stood in front of the platform waiting. We had hardly started to pray before he began to speak in tongues. He got healed and delivered, and he reprimanded the others from his village for not responding fast enough to the invitations for prayer. He reprimanded his older sister because he couldn't understand how one could be so dumb as to just sit there on the ground and not go forward when one could actually be healed!

The translator giggled so much at the old man's words, gestures, and style that I had to ask him to tell me what he was saying. We enjoyed seeing how this old man helped throughout the whole festival, and I often think of him. He was clothed in just a cloth around his loins and a bright yellow jacket from an aid/relief shipment. The jacket had the word "coach" written on the back and clung to his skinny, bare torso.

He was totally awesome, and I said at the end of the meetings that "all you have to do is follow your 'coach' here, and everything will be just fine." He was a constant example for every sermon and living proof that Jesus does miracles for someone who is hungry for them and believes that they will happen.

We baptized 101 newly saved people at the end of the festival. He slept down by the shore of the river because he wanted to be baptized first...and he was!

CHAPTER 19

# The Healing Touch

*We Will Study Luke 22:50-51*

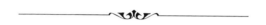

AT THE END OF JESUS' MINISTRY, in the garden of Gethsemane, a miracle took place that we so easily miss in our Bible reading because our thoughts are often taken up by details concerning the story of Jesus' death. Right when the temple guards were to arrest Jesus, right before He was sentenced to death by crucifixion, something happened, something quite remarkable.

One of the disciples took out his sword as if from nowhere. In a last desperate attempt to defend his Master, he cut off the right ear of one of the high priest's servants. It happened so fast, right in the middle of all the chaos of people shouting and fleeing and running to and fro. The whole arrest of Jesus stopped for a short moment when Jesus stretched out His hand and touched the bloody head and ear of the servant; immediately he was healed. The raw night air in Gethsemane was filled with the healing power of Jesus.

> *And one of them struck the servant of the high priest, cutting off his right ear. But Jesus answered, "No more of this!" And He touched the man's ear and healed him* (Luke 22:50-51).

A healing touch is something that we need to practice a whole lot more than what we do today. A hand that touches you gently on the neck or a soft brushing on the cheek can make a warmth flow through your whole body. I am not talking about romance or an erotic type of touch but instead a warm, pure, and loving touch.

There is healing and a deep secret in just this kind of touch. I have received this myself and have been able to pass it on as well. I know that what is written in this passage about Jesus is about a physical healing, but I also know that this servant could never forget the touch of Jesus or His calm eyes in the moment of this miracle.

I met my sister Anna, who is two years younger than me, in a school auditorium after a sweaty and wild meeting in Sweden. Anna had come together with two of my younger sisters and mother to listen to me and a team from Mission SOS speak. Both Anna and I had gone through quite a lot of suffering and darkness in our childhood. We looked at each other, and our eyes filled with tears. No words needed to be said. We understood each other so well. Suddenly Anna grabbed me and gave me a long, hard hug. I don't know how long that hug lasted, but it was a healing touch. It was an acknowledgment, an encouragement, an "I believe in you, Johannes" touch.

Anna is a midwife and is married with three children; I am a preacher, married with two children. We have long since left home and are grown-ups now, but oh, how I needed that hug right then and there. I felt such a warmth and felt so whole on the inside after quite a tough time with lots of misunderstandings around my ministry here in Sweden. I know that Anna, who is a devout Christian woman, was able to administer a healing to my soul from Jesus. Anna was probably not even aware of what happened to me on the inside, but I know that God was. I will never, ever forget that hug.

It happens sometimes that I just have to go down and hug someone who is standing in the line for salvation at a large festival meeting. Once, when I put my arms around a tough Pakistani guy and then put my right hand through his beard on his left cheek, he broke down and started to cry like a baby. He was healed. He got a much-needed inner healing. I knew that something from Jesus had flowed from me to him in that moment!

CHAPTER 20

# A New Thought

*We Will Study John 5:1-17*

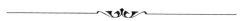

During the time of Jesus, right inside the Sheep Gate in Jerusalem, there was a pool called Bethesda. Ruins from this pool are still left today, and there are large archaeological digs in connection to this place. I have been there many times.

The pool was surrounded by five covered colonnades; many who were sick, blind, lame, and crippled would lay there. The place was well-known because of a strange spiritual phenomenon. The notorious place had its own legend that claimed that at certain times an angel would come down and stir up the water, and the one who first got into the water would be free from his ailment and immediately healed. It didn't really say if the angel was seen or not, but from this passage in the Bible, we know that the water was stirred from time to time. That is why there were many sick and lame lying there waiting for their turn.

Here Jesus met a lame man who had been sick for 38 years. He also was waiting for the healing stir of the water and had camped out by the side of the pool so as not to miss the next opportunity when it came. Up until now, someone had always made it in before him. Because of his sickness, it took too long for him to get into the water when it started moving. What a tragic healing lottery!

The lame man explained this to Jesus, who had just asked him if he really wanted to be well (see John 5:1-7). What a rude question to ask a man who had waited so long! The man had built his whole life around and had waited every waking moment for this miracle. But as usual, Jesus' question was justified.

The problem was that the man was completely stuck in his way of thinking of how the miracle should take place. According to him, it was supposed to happen in a certain way: *The angel will stir up the water—the water will start moving—I need to get into the water first....* He was completely blocked in this way of thinking: *This is how a miracle will take place. This is the method of healing I believe in.*

It is not so different from how people think today either, I should add. There are many people who need to have a new thought from time to time—at least once every 30 years anyway!

Then it happened: *"Jesus said to him, 'Get up! Pick up your mat and walk.' At once the man was cured; he picked up his mat and walked"* (John 5:8-9).

A completely new and revolutionary thought came into the lame man's head after 38 years: *And one can do it this way too! If I can just stand up, take my mat, and walk, then well, why not?! If you have said it, Jesus, then I will do it.* And he did.

I hear these same claims so often among people who have just received a miracle. They ask, "Was it that simple?!" Yes, imagine that it is just that easy!

CHAPTER 21

# Clay on the Eyes

*We Will Study John Chapter 9*

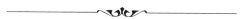

JESUS AND HIS DISCIPLES MET A BEGGAR who had been blind from birth. Jesus said to His disciples something that was well suited for the occasion—He said that He is the light of the world. Then something new happened. Yes, again, it was not the first time He had gotten the disciples to stare at Him with wide eyes wondering. It was exciting to follow Jesus!

> *Having said this, He spit on the ground, made some mud with the saliva, and put it on the man's eyes. "Go," He told him, "wash in the Pool of Siloam" (this word means Sent). So the man went and washed, and came home seeing* (John 9:6-7).

Saliva and dirt made clay or a type of healing dough that was laid on the eyes, and after an eyewash the man who had been blind his whole life could see!

Who could understand this? It was just another incredible miracle from Jesus! Sound judgment and intellect just stand with jaws wide open when God does a miracle.

This passage of Scripture has taught me that it wasn't really the beggar who was blind and had clay on his eyes; it was the religious elite who refused to believe the miracle. When the beggar came back from the Pool of Siloam seeing with perfect vision, it naturally caused confusion among those who knew him from before. Some said that it was him, and others said no, it was just someone who looked like him. Of course, he said, "It is me!" (See John 9:8-9.)

It was the Sabbath that day, and now someone had been healed. The religious leaders thought that was terrible, because it must have meant that someone had performed some kind of labor. The beggar explained, very clearly, what had happened to the religious leaders, the elite and orthodox Pharisees. Despite this, they did not believe him. They interviewed his parents, who confirmed that it was their son and that he had been born blind. The parents had no idea as to how he could now see. The religious leaders got angry and said to the beggar, "Give glory to God. We know this man is a sinner" (John 9:24).

You know, it is really irritating when someone you have judged is actually "for real." When they noticed that He wasn't the quack they thought He was, but really sent from God Most High, what could they do? This miracle was just too good to explain away. The beggar said it so wonderfully: *"Whether He is a sinner or not, I don't know. One thing I do know. I was blind but now I see!"* (John 9:25).

The religious elite, in whatever guise they showed up, always had a habit of running off that which they could not get a grip on or that which was too strong for them. And that was exactly what they did with the beggar. They threw him out with some harsh words saying that he was completely born in sin. They said that he should not try to teach them anything because they already had all the answers to all the questions. The religious elite have always had a hard time believing and usually would not allow themselves to be convinced that they were wrong, even if the evidence lined up in a long row against them. If they were to confess to being wrong, then their whole world would come crashing down on them.

*"Jesus said, 'For judgment I have come into this world, so that the blind will see and those who see will become blind'"* (John 9:39). Some Pharisees heard Him say this and asked, "Are we also blind?" Jesus answered quickly, *"If you were blind, you would not be guilty of sin; but now that you claim you can see, your guilt remains"* (John 9:41). The religious elite have always had clay on their eyes....

Not so long ago, our missionary Lisa Hjertberg became part of a fantastic miracle. She was in a poor Turkish/Gypsy village in southern Bulgaria. A 12-year-old girl came forward and explained that she couldn't see very well. In order to find out how bad her situation was, Lisa backed up approximately three meters and held up some fingers. The girl could not count how many fingers she held up.

Lisa then laid her hands on the girl's eyes and started to pray. The Holy Spirit then whispered in Lisa's ear: "Do like Jesus did; mix your saliva with some dirt, make a clay dough, and put it on her eyes." Lisa was surrounded by Muslims and hesitated a little. First she just put some saliva on the girl's eyes, but then felt that she could not ask the girl if she had been healed because she knew that she hadn't really obeyed what the Holy Spirit had told her to do. Lisa then made her decision. While the little girl probably wondered what she was up to, Lisa knelt down to the ground, mixed her saliva with the dirt, and then daubed it on the little girl's eyes. Then she prayed in the name of Jesus that the girl would completely receive her sight back. Immediately the healing power of God came!

After the prayer, the girl said that she could see well, but Lisa wanted to be completely sure that Jesus had done a miracle. She then did a new test; she now went at least ten meters back. This time the girl could see and count the number of fingers she was holding up without any problem!

CHAPTER 22

# Healing of the Soul

*We Will Study John 21:1-17*

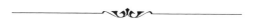

ONE OF THE MOST BEAUTIFUL STORIES IN THE Gospels, in my opinion, is found in the last chapter of the Gospel of John. It is a precious story of the restoration of a relationship, and the reinstated confidence of Jesus in a disciple who had failed. A second chance after a failure is what many people need. Jesus had been sentenced to death, died, and been buried. But now He had risen from the dead and was alive again, just like He had said would happen.

Simon Peter betrayed Jesus by denying that he even knew Him when the guards came to the garden of Gethsemane to imprison Him. It was a great betrayal for Peter, three times in a row, and he was now a broken man. Peter had betrayed the One he loved most on this earth—the One he had followed for more than three years, with whom he had witnessed so many signs and wonders. Peter loved Jesus' style, humor, straightforwardness, radicalism, and His love for people...but everything was over now. Peter, who had so boldly and confidently promised to never leave or fail Jesus, in the end, did just that.

Well, well...Peter fled back to his old profession, back to his old way of life. He returned to the fishing boat with its nets and gear and everything else that was comfortable and familiar to him there by the Sea of Galilee where he had grown up. Together with six of the twelve disciples, Peter cast out to sea and fished all night, but to no avail; they caught nothing.

Early the next morning, as they were steering the boat toward the shore, they saw a man, standing on the shore, who bore the resemblance of someone they knew. They seemed to recognize His silhouette, but it was still too far off to tell who it was for sure. It could not possibly be Him... The man was calling out to them, asking if they had caught anything to eat. When they answered no, He told them to put out the nets on the right side of the boat. They obeyed, and immediately caught a large amount of fish. They then realized who the man was!

Peter recognized this scenario from the very first day he had met the Master. The same thing had happened then also. They had caught an enormous amount of fish, and after that Peter decided to leave everything and follow Jesus.

Now, John said slightly out of breath and excitedly to Peter, *"It is the Lord!"* (John 21:7). Peter then jumped into the water and ran up the shore onto dry land, despite that they were almost there anyway. Peter responded spontaneously to the love and longing he had for Jesus. When he reached land, and they had pulled the boat that was overflowing with fish onto the shore, Peter then became shy and pensive. He was unusually quiet and reserved for his personality.

Peter felt his betrayal burn in his chest. He had a big knot in his stomach and tears started to well up in his eyes. He sat down broken and crushed next to the simmering coals left from the campfire that Jesus had lit during the night.

He understood that Jesus had probably slept there on the shore. At least He had waited a long while for them—yes, for him...Jesus had made breakfast: freshly grilled fish and fresh bread. Peter sat quietly, together with the others, and tried to eat. He couldn't seem to get much down. The fish and bread seemed to stick in his throat, like when you are eating just to be polite and don't dare say, "No thank you." Jesus just sat there, calm, cool, and collected as usual, and poked the fire with a stick.

Suddenly the silence was broken by a question. Jesus looked Peter straight in the eyes and said, *"Simon son of John, do you truly love Me more than these?"* Peter's tears started to run down his cheeks; he didn't dare look Jesus in the eyes but answered with a small voice: *"Yes, Lord, You know that I love You."* Now Jesus said some remarkable words: *"Feed My lambs"* (John 21:15). *What does He mean?* Peter must have thought to himself. *It's over. I am happy just to sit here and eat breakfast with Him. I don't deserve the ministry of a shepherd.* Now Jesus asked him again: *"Simon son of John, do you truly love Me?"* Now Peter really had to fight off the tears when he answered with a quivering voice: *"Yes, Lord, You know that I love You."* Jesus said the remarkable words again, only clearer and more emphatically this time: *"Take care of My sheep"* (John 21:16).

Peter must have thought: *Jesus is talking to me as if nothing has happened. I have betrayed Him; I was a coward and fled. I am not worthy to be anyone's shepherd at all. Jesus knows everything, and even so He does not condemn me. He must know that if I could only turn back the hands of time I would.* Peter understood that Jesus knew that he was remorseful over what he had done and really just wanted the Master's forgiveness—nothing more. Peter started to understand that he had already received Jesus' forgiveness and that Jesus had not given up on him at all but had great plans for his future. Peter started to become a little hopeful sitting there in his slightly wet clothes in the hazy morning dew that was mixed with smoke from the campfire.

Then Jesus asked for the third time: *"Simon son of John, do you love Me?"* Now Peter completely broke down and wept deeply as he despairingly answered: *"Lord, You know all things; You know that I love You."* His internal monologue might have continued: *You know everything, everything; You know everything, Jesus. You know that I thought I was stronger than I was. You know that I have betrayed You, disgraced myself, and lost everything.* Jesus said calmly: *"Feed My sheep"* (John 21:17). His simple words communicated much more to Peter: "You are forgiven. I believe in you. You are restored, Peter."

The conversation continued through dawn that early morning as the sun rose over the Sea of Galilee. This was about the disciples' future, about continuing to follow Jesus with their focus intact and probably a lot of other things. Peter had now experienced healing of the soul and inner healing. For every time he had betrayed and denied Jesus, he had now told Him how much he loved Him.

No psychologist or therapist in the world could have done a better job than Jesus. No counselor could have found such a perfect place and situation for a restorative conversation as Jesus did that special morning. A new time had begun for Peter and all the rest of the disciples. This was a new start, a new sunrise, and a new day for Peter, John, and the others!

I was very broken when I, as a young adult, made the decision to follow Jesus and His course for my life. Drawing near to Jesus, meditating on the Word, and lots of praying in tongues have made me whole on the inside. Jesus, only Jesus, can heal the soul and give total inner healing!

## Chapter 23

# Mass Miracles

---

IN CHAPTERS 3 THROUGH 22, I HAVE PRIMARILY described the personal meeting between Jesus and one or two people. In some cases, I have also tried to paint a picture and teach from Jesus' meeting with a smaller group of people. But now, let's get in a helicopter and fly in over the miracle-hungry masses. We're going to look at Jesus' ministry from a higher perspective for just a moment.

Surprisingly often during His relatively short and intense time of ministry here on earth, which lasted only three and one half years, Jesus gathered very large crowds. Of course, it is hard to know exactly how many Jesus spoke to at one time, but the Gospels describe some of the magnitude.

He ministered without the powerful public address systems that we have today to help us to be heard in a large gathering. Jesus and His disciples inventively used nature's own amphitheaters and the natural acoustics and resonance effects of the sea and the mountains.

Tens of thousands of people were gathered several times, both in connection with the "feeding of the five thousand" and at other occasions. We read in the Gospel of Luke, for example: *"Meanwhile, when a crowd of many thousands had gathered, so that they were trampling on one another, Jesus began to speak"* (Luke 12:1a).

There is something extra special in the dynamics of a large crowd. To sit with 34,000 people and watch a soccer match in a stadium is fun. To listen to a great rock star singing in front of a swaying sea of people at the Stockholm stadium or at another packed sports arena is really one of the most fantastic Swedish summer experiences. But to be part of a "Signs and Wonders" festival, arranged by our Swedish missions organization called Mission SOS—*that* is something I would encourage everyone reading this book to do, before you throw in the towel! (Maria and I think that the SOS workers are the world's best team! We love you!) Mass meetings with Jesus as the star and artist, with signs and wonders as the big attraction—that is an experience that will produce memories for life!

When Jesus gathered the largest crowds, people came for specific reasons that I would like to mention briefly. There must have been a reason that so many people gathered, right?

### 1) *They came to hear Jesus preach!*

Literally, there was no one in all of Israel who could capture an audience, be so popular with the people, and at the same time be as down to earth as Jesus was. Jesus preached the Word directly from God to them, spoken exactly at the right time!

> *Yet the news about Him spread all the more, so that crowds of people came to hear Him and to be healed of their sicknesses* (Luke 5:15).

*"Consequently, faith comes from hearing the message, and the message is heard through the word of Christ"* (Rom. 10:17). It is when we preach the Word of God that people receive faith and receive healing for their bodies.

*"Then the disciples went out and preached everywhere, and the Lord worked with them and confirmed His word by the signs that accompanied it"* (Mark 16:20). When we preach the pure, straightforward Gospel, then God confirms His own Word.

### 2) They came to be healed by Jesus!

*For He had healed many, so that those with diseases were pushing forward to touch Him* (Mark 3:10).

As I mentioned earlier, in March 1999, Maria and I, together with a smaller team from Mission SOS and another evangelist couple from Sweden, held three healing conferences in Pakistan in the cities of Karachi, Lahore, and Islamabad (see Chapter 14). What incredible healing and delivering power we saw! We saw clubfeet shrink and legs that were twisted by polio straighten out again! The blind received their sight, the deaf could hear again, and people who were bound to wheelchairs for many years were running back and forth over the platform. Every evening the demon-possessed were taken to deliverance tents, which we usually call "demon clinics," where the evil spirits were commanded to leave their victims because of the powerful name of Jesus.

### 3) Jesus had the kind of love that you could not deny.

Jesus was not "exclusive"; He loved people, was down to earth, and lived in contact with others. He was full of empathy and had strong and genuine compassion. The apostle Paul wrote in one of his letters: *"If I have a faith that can move mountains, but have not love, I am nothing"* (1 Cor. 13:2).

When you pass by a beggar sitting on the sidewalk, with paralyzed legs, what do you feel in your heart? Do you just walk by completely unmoved and maybe throw a few coins in the jar being held out to you with a very dirty hand? What benefit does that have? We must love more than a quarter's worth in a beggar's jar or a compassionate smile given in passing on a shopping trip! What benefit do your pennies and your distorted smile have on this poor guy on the sidewalk? No, it takes a little more than that, and Jesus had more than just a little bit of comfort for the moment: *"When He saw the crowds, He had compassion on them, because they were harassed and helpless, like sheep without a shepherd"* (Matt. 9:36).

Without love in your heart for people who have never heard the Gospel, your faith is meaningless, a resounding cymbal that sounds awful (see 1 Cor. 13:1). It was the compassionate heart of Jesus, full to the brim with love, that met the lost crowd of people with life and health. Ask God for a new heart that beats in line with His! (See 1 John 4:19.)

### 4) *Jesus and His disciples were good organizers.*

Think of the incredible chaos that must have come with all these people. So many were being healed that many were pushing and shoving in order to get to where Jesus was. The demon-possessed were throwing themselves in front of Him. Yes, of course, it was sometimes tumultuous, but when it got out of hand, Jesus' disciples organized a boat for Him to get into so that He did not get crushed in the crowd (see Mark 3:9).

A big rock concert requires guards, hosts, and riot fences, and so does a miracle festival. In all large gatherings, organization and practical aid is needed.

Imagine the day of Pentecost, when three thousand people wanted to get baptized on the same day (see Acts 2:41). It is clear that the disciples who had been with Jesus so long knew what good organization was and had well-planned logistics.

After some years, a team of disciples becomes a well-greased machine; they are so in sync with each other that they can almost handle anything thrown at them. They move and act as disciplined as an army, if needed, and know how to use professional administration. They each know their part, their titles, and special tasks, and harmony rules even in the midst of the storm, in the midst of rock throwing and emergency alarms (the author is smiling at the memories).

It is written that before Jesus did one of His great food miracles, the disciples were given the task of administrating what was about to take place: *"Then Jesus directed them to have all the people sit down in groups on the green grass. So they sat down in groups of hundreds and fifties"* (Mark 6:39-40).

Yeah, try to do that yourself! Distribute food to 15 to 20 thousand people without a well-thought-out plan and functioning organization! Effectiveness and administration in a mass-miracle ministry require coworkers, anointed directly from Heaven, with those types of capabilities and talents.

### 5) Jesus had a good reputation and a good track record.

*At that very time Jesus cured many who had diseases, sicknesses and evil spirits, and gave sight to many who were blind. So He replied to the messengers,* **"Go back and report to John what you have seen and heard***: The blind receive sight, the lame walk, those who have leprosy are cured, the deaf hear, the dead are raised, and the good news is preached to the poor"* (Luke 7:21-22).

All of this was proof that Jesus was the Jews' Messiah. The prophecy from the Book of Isaiah had been fulfilled: *"Then will the eyes of the blind be opened and the ears of the deaf unstopped. Then will the lame leap like a deer, and the mute tongue shout for joy"* (Isa. 35:5-6b).

In the synagogue in Nazareth, Jesus Himself read out of the Book of Isaiah: *"The Spirit of the Lord is on Me, because He has anointed Me to preach good news to the poor. He has sent*

*Me to proclaim freedom for the prisoners and recovery of sight for the blind, to release the oppressed, to proclaim the year of the Lord's favor"* (Luke 4:18-19).

Mankind has always wanted proof. Miracles and healings were the signs that Jesus was the Savior, the Messiah. Peter preached on the day of Pentecost: *"Men of Israel, listen to this: Jesus of Nazareth was a man accredited by God to you by miracles, wonders and signs, which God did among you through Him, as you yourselves know"* (Acts 2:22).

Jesus had a reputation that spread like wildfire. Many times the people gathered around Jesus just because of His powerful reputation. Mass miracles in Jesus' ministry created amazement and astonishment among the people. Never before had so many sick people been healed at one occasion! It gave birth to thankfulness, and Jesus' desire to glorify the Father was fulfilled when the people praised and worshiped God:

> *Jesus left there and went along the Sea of Galilee. Then He went up on a mountainside and sat down.* **Great crowds** *came to Him, bringing the lame, the blind, the crippled, the mute and many others, and laid them at His feet; and He healed them.* **The people were amazed** *when they saw the mute speaking, the crippled made well, the lame walking and the blind seeing.* **And they praised the God of Israel** (Matthew 15:29-31).

## MIRACLE POWER

At the end of this chapter about Jesus' mass-miracle ministry, I must tell yet another story from our festival work in Mission SOS. The apostle Paul hit the point when he said, *"I will not venture to speak of anything except what Christ has accomplished through me in leading the Gentiles to obey God by what I have said and done—by the power of signs and miracles, through the power of the Spirit"* (Rom. 15:18-19a).

Children were dancing in the red dust in front of the festival platform at the end of a scorching hot and sweaty miracle meeting in southern Kenya. It was already late in the afternoon. The sun was starting to set, and the Kuria and Luoa people's worship was wild and captivating. We all—including 114 Swedes from Mission SOS and some 15,000 Africans—had a reason to celebrate because Jesus, the Son of the living God, had done miracles again! Great miracles! We were hoarse in our voices, euphorically happy, and consumed with thankfulness to God that we were alive and could sing on this warm afternoon in March 2004.

Suddenly we saw a little handicapped boy, 12 years of age, sit down on his rump in the dust, among the hundreds of wildly dancing and yelling children. Our attention was drawn to him like a magnet to metal, partially because he had such a surprised expression on his face but also because he was trying frantically to untie his specially made shoe. The shoe had a built-up sole and supporting braces from the ankles up to the knees with an iron ring just above the knee to hold everything in place. (An orthopedist would laugh at this evangelist's attempt to describe the brace, but anyway....) The boy's foot was deformed from birth, and his calf was crooked and bent.

In the middle of his clumsy attempt to dance together with all the other children in the festival rave, suddenly he had started to feel pain in his foot. The boy thought that there must be a rock in his shoe rubbing so hard against his foot that he just had to take the whole thing off. Now when he had taken off his shoe, he was astonished to find that his foot had become completely normal and his calf had straightened out! His foot was hurting because his foot did not fit in the specially made shoe any longer. He came running up the stairs to us on the platform with his brace in his hands; the shoe, support braces, leather straps, and iron rings were held up into the evening sun, while the boy was leaping and jumping around us. Almost everyone was celebrating. Some were crying and some were shaking their heads in quiet amazement with tears running down their cheeks. The miracle power from Jesus was there! The boy, who came from a Muslim home, said, "Your Jesus must have made me well!"

The joy knew no bounds when the children followed him home singing and laughing and handing over the foot brace to his shocked Muslim parents. The children were all talking at once, "He doesn't need this brace anymore. Jesus has made him well!"

I have seen it so many times, but I never get tired of it. There is nothing like the healing power of Jesus. He is risen; He is alive! I love to serve Him because He is so wonderful! It is said about Jesus: *"And the power of the Lord was present for Him to heal the sick"* (Luke 5:17b).

Once Jesus gathered people on a plain in Israel, and the physician Luke described the event for us: *"Who had come to hear Him and to be healed of their diseases. Those troubled by evil spirits were cured, and the people all tried to touch Him, because power was coming from Him and healing them all"* (Luke 6:18-19).

Miracle power from Jesus Himself is what the world needs more of. Usually this miracle power is the key to the demonic "padlock," which makes the satanic chains that have plagued people's lives fall to the ground. We must dare to preach the Gospel plain and simple, and cry out to God so that miracle power falls over all the unreached peoples now! We must bring closure to the great commission.

> *And this gospel of the kingdom will be preached in the whole world as a testimony to all nations, and then the end will come* (Matthew 24:14).

# Chapter 24

# Healing in the Book of Acts

Jesus left this earth with a last request to His disciples: to wait. Wait for what? Wait to be clothed with power from on high to be His witnesses in all the earth (see Acts 1:4-5,8). A few days later, on the day of Pentecost, they were baptized in the Holy Spirit and equipped to do the things that Jesus did—and more! *"I tell you the truth, anyone who has faith in Me will do what I have been doing. He will do even greater things than these..."* (John 14:12). In the Book of Acts, the first history book of the first church, we can, through the physician and author Luke, be part of a real adventure and miracle-discovery trip. Put your seat belt on because now it's starting to roll!

## Give What You Have

Just a few days after the early church's "birthday," Peter and his companions met the man who was carried out to beg in front of the gate called "Beautiful," right in front of the temple in Jerusalem. The man, who from birth had been paralyzed from his waist down, asked promptly for a gift when he saw they were about to walk by. (See Acts 3:2-3.) Peter, who now had the man's full attention, said to him: *"Silver or gold I do not have, but **what I have I give you**. In the name of Jesus Christ of Nazareth, walk"* (Acts 3:6). Then he took the man's hand and drew him up from the ground. Immediately the man stood upright, with full strength in his feet and ankles, and followed them both into the temple, walking and jumping and praising God.

When Peter saw the astonished and staring crowd who were filled with surprise over what had happened to the well-known, handicapped beggar, he asked them:

> *Men of Israel, why does this surprise you? Why do you stare at us as if by our own power or godliness we had made this man walk? The God of Abraham, Isaac and Jacob, the God of our fathers, has glorified His servant **Jesus**....By faith in the name of Jesus, this man whom you see and know was made strong. **It is Jesus' name** and the faith that comes through Him that has given this complete healing to him, as you can all see* (Acts 3:12-13,16).

Peter then preached the Gospel, and two thousand received Christ as a direct result of this remarkable and powerful miracle!

He who has a wallet filled with gold and silver knows that he need not be worried if someone asks him for money. He doesn't need to go and get help somewhere else, borrow from anyone, or even go to an ATM and withdraw money. He knows that what is in his wallet is his and that he can give it to anyone he chooses!

That which Peter had received was not money, but he, just like every Christian, had received the name of Jesus (see Acts 4:12), and he had confidence in the Holy Spirit! He knew that he didn't need to get some Christian leader with greater faith than he had when he went to help the lame man. What he had on the inside was enough! (See Acts 3:1-16.)

Walk with your head held high. *Be confident in what God has given you, and give what you have,* knowing that what you have is *the name of Jesus!*

### DARE TO BE AWARE OF YOUR AUTHORITY IN CHRIST!

Despite being forbidden to speak or preach in the name of Jesus and despite the persecution of the Christians, the apostles performed so many miracles that people everywhere were coming to faith in Jesus Christ. In Jerusalem, they were not able to stop the rumors of what was being said about the incredible miracles taking place! Massive amounts of people from the surrounding cities traveled there with their sick family members, relatives, and neighbors, in order to come in contact with this healing power. *"As a result, people brought the sick into the streets and laid them on beds and mats* **so that at least Peter's shadow might fall on some of them as he passed by**" (Acts 5:15). And all of them were healed!

Peter didn't lay his hands on every sick person who wanted his help, nor did he give them personal intercessory prayer, but at the very moment that Peter's shadow fell on people, they were made well! Peter knew his authority in Christ. He carried the miracle power within him, and he had a spirit that took over in every place that he came to! (See Acts 5:12-16.) Learn what authority you have in Christ, for you are His representative in the elevator, at your workplace, or in line at McDonald's. Take over the place with the Holy Spirit!

### THOSE WHO *HEAR* AND *SEE* BELIEVE!

When the members of the early church were dispersed and spread out as a result of hard persecution that broke out in Jerusalem, Philip, one of the practical helpers, came to a city called Samaria. He immediately started preaching Jesus to the inhabitants of the city. Demons started screaming out when they left the bodies of many of the listeners, and other people with visible sicknesses and disabilities were made well. There was great joy in the whole city. *"When the crowds heard Philip and saw the miraculous signs he did,* **they all paid close attention to what he said**" (Acts 8:6).

Philip preached Jesus to the people, but it says that they believed only after they had heard and seen the signs that took place. (See Acts 8:5-8.)

It is fantastic, of course, when someone is healed from a headache—and God always loves to heal all sicknesses—but one of the goals of a miracle is that it be a sign for people, so they can start to believe. The Word of God is always confirmed by signs! (See Mark 16:20.) Being healed from a headache is not anything anyone can hear or see. Expect great and visible miracles when you proclaim the Gospel message!

## THE HOLY SPIRIT IS NOT PREDICTABLE

After receiving a direct word from God, Ananias went to the house where Saul had been staying for the past three days, since the day he was made blind. Ananias came in, laid his hands on him, and informed Saul about the God who had met him on the road: *"The Lord—Jesus, who appeared to you on the road as you were coming here—has sent me so that you may see again and be* **filled with the Holy Spirit**" (Acts 9:17). Saul, who later received the name Paul, immediately received his sight back and was baptized! (See Acts 9:18.)

Many times we want to list the ways that God will meet a person and in what order everything should take place! But healing is just a part of the whole capacity of God. Often people will be saved and filled with the Holy Spirit at the same time they are healed! Don't be surprised when the young

Muslim with whom you are praying for healing starts to babble in tongues even though you have not even prayed the sinner's prayer yet! Healing, salvation, baptism, and baptism in the Holy Spirit go hand in hand! We work together with the Holy Spirit, and *He is not predictable, but He is sovereign!*

One of our missionaries tells about a similar experience during her first Jesus festival in Dire Dawa, Ethiopia, in the spring of 2005:

> During an "outreach," I was going to pray for a man who had explained in broken English that he had pain in his jaw or mouth. While I was praying that God would heal him, I suddenly heard that he started to make strange and funny noises. Suddenly, he screamed out, and then he started to speak in tongues and was crying at the same time. After having prayed together for a while, I asked him if he had experienced something like this before, but he just shook his head. He had been both healed and baptized in the Holy Spirit at the same time!

## CHALLENGE THEM TO ACT!

When Peter was on his way through a city called Lydda, a little northwest of Jerusalem, he met a man called Aeneas, who had been bedridden for eight years. Peter said to the lame man: *"Aeneas,* **Jesus Christ heals you. Get up and take care of your mat"** (Acts 9:34). Immediately, Aeneas acted on the words spoken to him by Peter, and when all of the inhabitants of this area heard of this key miracle, they repented and believed in Jesus Christ! (See Acts 9:32-35.)

The words of Peter breathed faith. He did not say to Aeneas that Jesus wanted to or would in the future heal him, but that Jesus would heal him *now*. After that, he spoke out a challenge and a command from the Holy Spirit: "Get up and take care of your mat." The man had not received any proof that he was healed, no change in his body had taken place yet—he might not even have had a "warm current" going through his body. The only thing he received was a word of faith and a heavenly challenge. His *acting* in faith led to a fantastic miracle in his body! When you pray for someone for healing in the name of Jesus, challenge them to act in faith!

One of my SOS missionaries at our base in Bulgaria tells how she acted in faith and was healed:

> I have been allergic to dogs since I was four or five years old. My throat always started to itch and scratch, and then I started to sneeze if I was in the same room as a dog. After a teaching about healing at SOS Mission Bible College, we prayed for each other, and I wanted to test my healing. I got in a car, together with one of my classmate's long-haired German shepherds, and petted him and rubbed my nose in his fur. I didn't have a reaction at all as I normally would have had before, and now I no longer need to take my allergy medicine!

## Follow the Intuition of Your Spirit!

The apostle Paul and his partner Barnabas were preaching the Gospel in Lystra, a city in what today is southern Turkey. Paul fixed his eyes on a man who had not been able to walk since birth and was now among the crowd listening to Paul preach. When Paul *saw* that the lame man had *faith* to be healed, he said with a loud voice: *"Stand up on your feet!"* (Acts 14:10). At that, the man jumped up and began to walk! (See Acts 14:8-10.)

Paul sought eye contact with the man because he wanted to see if he had faith to be made well. When he saw the man's faith, he immediately led this man to healing!

Paul used the sensitivity and intuition that is like a tool in every man and woman's spirit. The Holy Spirit speaks and gives us impulses through our spirit. The fact that Paul dared to act on his spirit's intuition, and saw the man's faith, was the key to this miracle happening. It was a clear sign for everyone in that place! Dare to follow your spirit's intuition completely when you pray for the sick!

## Carry the Miracle Power With You!

During one of his mission trips, Paul came to the city of Ephesus. Here a lot of unusual miracles happened through his hands. When the city's inhabitants took home clothes and pieces of cloth that had been in contact with Paul's skin and placed them on the sick family members, the sick were healed and the demon-possessed were made free! (See Acts 19:11-12.)

Paul's faith led to an authority and faith for healing that took its expression physically! He carried the miracle power in him! Start carrying the miracle power in you too!

In February 1997, I was visiting the Masai people in southern Kenya, right on the border of the national park Masai Mara. A lot of people gathered around when the warriors came, in their red cloaks with their large families and herds of cattle. We did like Paul and handed out many "prayer cloths"—clothes, shawls, and handkerchiefs that we had laid our hands on and prayed over.

Approximately two months after we had arrived home, we received via mail many reports of healing from one of the local Masai pastors who worked with the follow-up. Approximately 1,400 people in the area had been healed through these pieces of clothing and handkerchiefs when taken home to the sick! After the power of Jesus had healed one sick body, the piece of clothing or cloth was then taken to another family, and so on.

The piece of cloth or clothing was a physical, substantial point of contact for faith in Jesus. The prayer cloths did not heal in and of themselves; the power in Jesus' blood and wounds, which was now in the prayer cloths, healed them. The prayer cloth can be a "carrier," or a pipeline for the power of Jesus. Blood cancer and diabetes—and yes, even deafness and blindness—were reported to have been healed, according to the compilation of the report.

During a festival organized by Mission SOS in a slum area in Ecuador in July 2001, a woman took home a handkerchief that we had prayed over. She had a tumor in her stomach. In faith that Jesus would heal her, she slept with the handkerchief on her stomach. The next day, she went to her doctor, and he did a new ultrasound examination. The tumor that was visible on the last ultrasound was now no longer there! Healed without an operation, the woman now had two ultrasound pictures to show—one with the tumor very visible, and the second with absolutely no tumor there! She had her miracle documented by medical doctors, and the next evening she happily stood on the platform. She shared her "story" and waved the documented proof in the air. Need I say that after that a healing explosion followed?!

## Ask God for Key Miracles!

On Paul's trip to Rome, his ship was wrecked in a violent storm. Despite that, all the passengers on board were saved and washed up onto shore on the island of Melita or Malta. The most prominent man on the island was a man called Publius, who received them as his guests. (See Acts 28:1-7.)

No one on the island had yet heard the Gospel, but at the same time Paul came to the island, Publius' father was sick with high fever and diarrhea. When the father was made well through Paul's prayers and his laying on of hands, the inhabitants of the island started to seek Paul for healing, and many were healed from their sicknesses! (See Acts 28:8-10.)

Paul landed totally unexpectedly on an island that was completely unreached by the Gospel. Through God's leading, he became friends with the island's most prominent man, whose father was miraculously healed! What happened was a key miracle!

A key miracle is one that unlocks the door to other healings and miracles; it is always followed by a wave of miracles and conversions. The fact that Publius' father was healed led to the whole island opening themselves up for Jesus and His servant Paul! (See Acts 28:8-9.) Ask God for key miracles!

In November 1997, I preached for some former head-hunting tribes on the island of Luzon in the northern Philippines. We visited the Ilongot and Igorot tribes in a paradise-like jungle of coconut trees. We gathered around a stage on a basketball court in a small village. On this cement stage in the middle of the wilderness, a team that I just happened to be leading was singing, dancing, and preaching for five days. Many people crowded around, and one evening, a woman who had been blind for 24 years could suddenly see the light from the spotlights. She cried out in Tagalog, her tribal language, "I see the light!"

That evening a healing process started in her eyes. I don't know what state her eyesight is in now, or if she got a complete healing later. Naturally, I want to believe that a complete healing took place; it usually does once the healing process has been started.

This key miracle opened the door to other miracles and a miracle explosion took place after that. The deaf received their hearing, and crutches were thrown away! Key miracles work even in this modern day and age!

CHAPTER 25

# Quotes From the Early Church Fathers About Healing

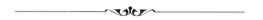

IN THIS CHAPTER, I WANT TO DISCUSS BRIEFLY what the early Christians thought and reasoned in regard to healing. Personally, I think that early church history provides fantastic reading material. (By early church history, I mean the first four hundred years after the Book of Acts—i.e., from the middle of A.D. 60 to A.D. 450.)

Theologians and apologists were then against Greek mythology, philosophy, and a stench of gnosticism that existed among the disciples. These people's life stories are almost a direct continuation of the Book of Acts. The early church and the first Christian leaders' self-sacrificing convictions and relentless commitment to their master Jesus is extremely fascinating.

To read about them is both humbling and inspiring. We will now meditate on a few quotes from some of those who took over the leadership in the churches, in the area of the Mediterranean Sea, after the apostles Peter and Paul both died as martyrs.

Jesus' apostles trained their disciples just like Jesus did: to conquer and take over the whole world for the Kingdom of God. About the same time that the Book of Acts ended, the persecution of Christians increased during Emperor Nero's reign. More and more Christians died as martyrs, happy and proud to suffer for Jesus.

The early Church spoke about three baptisms: baptism in water, baptism in fire, and baptism in blood (i.e., the martyr's death). When the Roman and Jewish leaders tried to wipe out the young Christian Church, the effects of the persecution had the opposite effect. The churches grew, and the Gospel spread like wildfire over large areas.

Apparitions of angels, deliverances from demons, and healings were very common—yes, actually ordinary, everyday happenings for the first generation of Christians. For several hundred years after the day of Pentecost, the miracles and signs continued to be a distinguishing feature for those who believed in Jesus Christ.

The early Church's first heroes can teach us a lot. We need to be smitten with their attitude and view of healing, at the same time enjoying their simple and raw faith and their refusal to compromise. Just remember that when we read these quotes, it is interesting reading, but absolutely not equal to that which is written in the Bible.

**The Shepherd of Hermas** was from Rome. He was a former slave of Jewish origin who was a Christian. At the end of the first century he wrote this: "He who knows that someone has a sickness and does not deliver him from it, commits a great sin and is guilty of his blood."

Radical? Oh yes, very much so. The Shepherd of Hermas saw it as an obligation not only to pray for all the sick but also to heal them. Today we as Christians can sometimes be satisfied with just praying for the sick person, even if nothing happens. Or maybe we are satisfied with the sick person being touched in his soul, despite the fact that the pain and suffering from the sickness is still there. The Shepherd of Hermas meant that we as Christians had received power, and with it...responsibility.

Let me give you two simple, everyday stories of how healing is given in a poor village in southern Bulgaria. A woman came up to one of our SOS missionaries and asked for prayer because she had pain in her shoulder. When the missionary took hold of her arm and lifted it carefully up over her head, the woman grimaced from the pain. The missionary lowered her arm and laid her hands on the woman, praying a short prayer in the name of Jesus. Then she took hold of the arm again and lifted it up high. The total amazement in the woman's eyes quickly changed to joy and relief. She was healed even without realizing it.

In the same village, there was a little girl who had never been able to move one of her arms. Another missionary in the same team prayed for this cute, little, dark-haired girl named Jifka. When she had finished praying, she had to work hard to convince the little girl she should try to move her fingers.

The missionary noticed that the girl could move her small fingers more and more every second that went by. After a few minutes, the little girl was able to stretch her arm straight up into the air, which she had never been able to do before in her six years of life.

The mother standing beside them had tears running down her cheeks. What a day of joy it was for that family! How would their day have ended if the missionary had just been satisfied with simply praying for the little girl, hoping that she maybe felt a little warm and fuzzy on the inside?

For the first Christians, there was no Christianity without deliverance from demons and healing.

One of the early church fathers, **Justinius the Martyr** (A.D. 100–165), said, "Christians heal people in the name of Jesus and cast out demons and all other kinds of evil spirits."

Quite obvious, huh?! He doesn't write, "Some Christians heal the sick." Nor does he say, "Christians can heal." If you are a Christian, then you heal the sick—it is as simple as that! Justinius was one of many early church fathers who suffered a martyr's death. He wrote a letter to the Christian-hating Emperor Marcus Aurelius and was quickly sentenced to death.

At the same time that Christianity grew and spread very quickly, different kinds of false teachings popped up, including messages that stood up against the true Gospel. Teachers and preachers came and taught their own revelations, in contrast to the words of the apostles. This led unstable disciples away from the truth. But many apologists (i.e., defenders of Christianity) rose up and fought for the pure and true Gospel message.

One of them was **Irenaeus**. He was a disciple of Polycarp, who was a disciple of John—one of Jesus' disciples! He wrote a whole book against these erroneous teachings. His answer to how one could recognize truth from untruth was simple: see if they heal people or not. He elaborated on this point in his book *Against Heresies*: "The heretics could not perform miracles of healing, which the Christians could do." The proof that they were not true followers of Christ was that "they didn't have access to the power of God and could not heal."

Quite simple, isn't it? If people are healed, then that means that God gives them a green light. You can then sit back, relax, and listen to their teaching because they are speaking the truth. If you do not see any signs and wonders, you should be careful.

Irenaeus also said: "The Lord raised the dead, and the apostles did it through prayer, and it has often happened in the brotherhood if it has been necessary. When the whole church at one place has bombarded heaven with prayer and much fasting, then the spirit of the dead person has returned as a result of the prayers of the righteous."

At the beginning of year A.D. 200, there was severe persecution against the Christians in northern Africa, and many Christians were martyred. **Origenes** was the oldest of six children, and his father was among them who were martyred. Origenes understood what was about to happen and wanted to follow his father into death. Had his mother not hidden his clothes that day, the Church would have lost one of its greatest thinkers and theologians of all time.

Origenes said about Christianity in general: "The Christians cast out many evil spirits and perform healings; I have witnessed many of these myself."

Once again, we see that it is a distinguishing feature and quite obvious that Christians heal the sick. Origenes also mentioned psychological healing and healing of the soul in his writings. He said, "I have also seen many people delivered from accidents, from mental problems, craziness and countless sicknesses that could not be healed by people or by a devil."

"Jesus' name can still take away mental sicknesses in people's minds, cast out demons, and take away sicknesses. It also produces an incredibly humble spirit and a totally changed character." We see in this quote from Origenes that it was very clear that Christian healings do not include only physical miracles. Healing of the soul and the mind were very common in the early Church. There are no impossible cases—Jesus heals all different kinds of sicknesses.

"Up to this time, those who God chooses have been healed in His name. This fact shows the authenticity in Jesus' ministry." To pray for the sick in the name of Jesus is to preach, he says here. In what way can you more clearly prove that Jesus is the Son of God than to heal the sick in His name? Every time we lay our hands on someone and pray for him in the name of Jesus, we give our Master an opportunity to prove that He is true. After Origenes had lived a long life, he died from complications of having been tortured and imprisoned for the sake of his Master and Savior, Jesus.

Let me give you one last quote. It was written by **Arnobius** in the year A.D. 350:

> Through His power, He not only did these miraculous deeds...but He has also allowed many others to try to do them by using His name....He chose fishermen, carpenters, farmers, and other uneducated people, so that they, sent to different countries, would perform all these miracles without fraud or any other kind of aid or means.

Isn't it wonderful that Jesus gives the right to use His name to simple people like us, so that we can go to different countries and without cheating or other aid do the work of Jesus? I love my Jesus for this!

Let me end this book's last chapter with a healing and deliverance story from the 21st century and from my own walk with Jesus.

In July 2001, I was in Ecuador, South America, in a large, outdoor arena in a slum area. I was preaching when right in the middle of my sermon I started to speak in tongues. I immediately felt that it was a prophetic language. I knew already while I was speaking in tongues who the heavenly message was directed to, and I pointed to a large man in the crowd among the thousands of listeners.

When God finally came with the interpretation, it revealed a sharp message that God knew about the physical abuse, unfaithfulness, lies, and hate—but that God now wanted to set him free! It was very detailed information.

The man fell down to the ground screaming as the demons started to leave his body; among other things were spirits of violence and a spirit of lust. He said after the meeting that he had wanted to kill me when I had revealed his perverse and hard lifestyle so brutally and frankly from the platform. Just when he thought of running forward to assault me, he was thrown to the ground by a strong force, and invisible hands held him pressed against the pavement. He couldn't move, but could only scream when the demons were leaving his body.

A little bit later he tearfully asked Jesus for forgiveness for his dirty lifestyle and became a new creature in Christ. The day after, he came with vegetables, meat, and other food. He wanted to thank me and the team because now his wife and children had also forgiven him. Naturally we said:

"Thank Jesus!"

The man was so thankful! Prophetic messages in tongues can be very powerful!

I hope that you as the reader will start to demonstrate the love of Jesus through His healing power wherever you go after reading this simple book. That has been my prayer while writing these chapters: Let the healing power of Jesus reach out to every sick person that has not yet received his or her miracle and let Jesus' healing ministry multiply.

Thank you for taking time to read a simple missionary and evangelist's attempt to teach. I pray for you as a reader that you will make more discoveries and experiences and receive more light on this every day. I am not finished yet, and I hope you are not either.

Bow your knee now and pray humbly to the God of the Bible that the Holy Spirit's power will start working through your life when you start using the wonderful and powerful name of Jesus. The book does not end here—it continues to be written by both you and me until Jesus returns!

# Epilogue

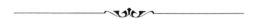

*Jesus did many other things as well. If every one of them were written down, I suppose that even the whole world would not have room for the books that would be written* (John 21:25).

THERE IS, OF COURSE, MUCH MORE TO BE SAID on the subject of healing in the Bible; there are also customs of healing that I have not touched on at all in this book. One very common practice in Christian circles, for example, is to "anoint the sick person with oil." Even though the Word says that the disciples did this (see Mark 6:13), it doesn't say anywhere that Jesus used oil to anoint people when He was healing them. James, the Lord's brother, encourages us to do this in addition to praying in faith (see James 5:14). That is why I have chosen to leave out that method, instead concentrating more specifically on Jesus' healing ministry.

It is naturally, absolutely, biblical to anoint the sick with oil. The oil is for us both a physical and practical picture of healing ointment and the Holy Spirit, who helps our faith and makes our prayers more specific.

We often anoint the sick with oil in Mission SOS's festivals and services with great success. The disciples were encouraged by Jesus to do greater miracles than what He Himself had done: *"I tell you the truth, anyone who has faith in Me will do what I have been doing. He will do even greater things than these, because I am going to the Father"* (John 14:12). After Jesus' death and resurrection, this is exactly what happened with Jesus' disciples, and it has continued even into our modern day through ordinary disciples all over the world.

The following are some stories of healing from our missionaries and coworkers. It is their uncensored, unembellished, and handwritten stories that are related. It is wonderful reading and just the tip of the iceberg from our archives. Hold on!

# References

- Bercot, David W. *A Dictionary of Early Christian Beliefs*. Peabody, MA: Hendrickson Publishers, 1998.
- Gonzalez, Justo. *The Story of Christianity*. Vol. 1. San Fransisco: Harper & Row, 1984.
- Halldorf, Peter. *21 Kyrkofäder (21 Church Fathers)*. Smedjebacken: Cordia, 2000.
- *Kyrkohistoria (Church History)*. Skellefteå: Eusebios, Artos, 1999.
- Mursell, Gordon. *Kristen Spiritualitet (Christian Spirituality)*. Singapore: Libris, 2006.

# Healing Testimonies and Photographs

# The Twisted Legs Straightened Out

There was total excitement that evening in April 2005, in Dire Dawa, Ethiopia, where the festival was taking place. I stood and watched as hundreds of people ran forward to the stage to receive that which the man on the stage had spoken about: a healing, a miracle from Jesus!

A couple thousand people had been saved during the week! After having prayed for a blind man who had received his sight and a few deaf people who had received hearing, I now wiped the sweat from my brow and looked for the next person who was in need of God's healing touch. Suddenly, a mother with a little girl in her arms came up to my friend and me. The girl had some form of autism. It was hard to make eye contact with the girl—she seemed like she was somewhere else—and her legs were completely twisted. She had never been able to walk; her mother had to carry her everywhere.

People all around us also saw the girl and were eagerly watching to see if God really could heal someone so gravely handicapped. My friend and I laid our hands on her and started to cry out to God for a miracle. We prayed for quite some time, but nothing happened. We then called two more friends to come and help us pray for the little girl. She sat on one of their laps, while I held firmly to one of her legs, my friend grabbed the other leg, and the fourth stood in front of us. We completely cried out to God for this little girl's healing. Nothing happened. We came to a point where we looked at each other and felt a kind of hopelessness, but we quickly shook it off and looked at each other even more desperately than before!

Naturally this little girl should be able to play just like all the other children; it was exactly what God wanted! When we cried out to God and commanded the legs to be well in the name of Jesus, it happened! Both of the girl's legs shook and straightened out while I was holding her in my hands! God is the same, yesterday, today, and forever!

Sarah Kindholm

# Free From Joint Pain and Gluten Allergy

During a campaign in Växjö, Sweden, in the fall of 2002, I prayed for a woman who suffered from fibromyalgia, pain in her shoulder joints, and a gluten allergy. As a result, she could not lift her arms higher than shoulder height or eat bread baked with regular flour. Her gluten allergy was so serious that if she sliced her bread with the same knife used to slice regular bread, she would get serious stomach pains.

That evening, I prayed a prayer in faith and desperation to God. Quite soon afterward, she started to swing her arms around, crying. I asked her carefully what had happened, and she said that she could no longer feel any pain! That very moment I was filled with even more faith, so I said to her that I thought God had also healed her from her gluten allergy!

That very evening, after the meeting, she went and bought a hotdog with normal white bread, and she ate it. Then she sat up half the night waiting to see if she would get pain in her stomach—but she felt nothing. The stomach pain never came! The day after that, I ran into her again, now with bread crumbs on her face, a paper bag filled with normal wheat bread, and a huge smile on her face; she was completely healed!

Daniel Elvelyck

# "I Felt How the Boil Disappeared"

He was a bearded, middle-aged man with worn hands. Surely he had worked hard during most of his lifetime. His clothes were dirty and torn. But there was something in his eyes, a hope that Jesus would do a miracle.

Part of the team and I sat on the edge of the stage in a church in Bulgaria, in the city of Pazardzik, in April of 2002. We were going to pray for the sick when this man suddenly stood in front of me. I asked him what he wanted and what I should pray for. He answered that it was not prayer for himself that he wanted but prayer for his son. I didn't see the boy because there were so many people crowding around, but the man lifted him up to me and pointed to a boil on his neck. It was as big as a ping pong ball. I thought to myself: *What if this is cancer or something else more serious? Good thing it is not me doing the healing.*

I was overwhelmed with compassion for this little two-year-old boy. I sat him on my knee, put my hand on the boil, and started to pray a very simple prayer. I just said, "Jesus, I ask you to make this little boy well so that he can live a happy and normal life."

Suddenly I felt how the boil started to disappear. I almost didn't believe it was true. I had hardly finished praying before the boil was gone. The boy just looked at me with his big, beautiful, dark eyes, while his father both cried and rejoiced at the same time when he saw what had happened. His hope had been fulfilled, and the father and son could leave that place knowing that Jesus had done a miracle for them!

Samuel Willkander

# Healing on the Commuter Train, Salvation on the Train Platform

I was on my way home from getting vaccinated in downtown Stockholm. On the commuter train back to Märsta, I was telling my friends how I had gotten saved and how my life was totally transformed. They had, of course, heard the story thousands of times, but it wasn't for them I was telling it but for all the other people that were sitting around us. After a while, I saw that there was a girl beside me with crutches. I asked her what had happened. She explained that she had injured her knee and that it was filled with fluid; the doctors didn't really know what was wrong. I asked her if she had heard what I was telling my friends about, and she said that she had. So I asked her if I could pray for her knee.

"Yes," she said, a little shyly.

So I started to pray. People around us cleared their throats to show their contempt for what I was doing, but I continued to pray. The train stopped, and everyone rushed out to the platform.

"Test your knee now," I said.

She carefully took a few steps with her crutches and then put them down and walked. She felt a little better. Before the prayer, she said that she hadn't been able to walk at all without her crutches; it was just too painful. I told her that she should test her healing by trying to walk completely without crutches. She tried again, and she walked perfectly without them. Her face in total shock, the girl told us that she wanted what we had. So my former girlfriend, now my wonderful wife, led her to Jesus in a prayer of salvation right there on the train platform. The tears ran down her cheeks as she said:

"I have never felt this way before."

Three days later I saw her come running toward me. Jesus had done a miracle!

Marcus Johnsen

# Third Time's the Charm

I was on a team mission trip to Harar, Ethiopia, in 2006. In the evenings, we had big festival meetings where we prayed for people who were sick.

A man came up to me and said that he was deaf in one ear and that he wanted me to pray for him. So I laid my hands on him and started to pray for him in the name of Jesus. Nothing happened, so I put my hands on him again and prayed one more time. He started to hear better, but he still was not 100 percent well in his ear, so I prayed for him a third time. This time Jesus opened his ears; he was totally and completely made well. I then led this man to salvation and the baptism in the Holy Spirit.

Oscar Liljemark

# The Spirit of Sickness Left Her

One afternoon in the southern part of Bulgaria, a little girl was standing right in front of me. Clothed in a dirty, red top, she looked up at me with her big brown eyes. Through the translator, I found out that she had a problem with her eyes—she could see, but very dimly and badly. I squatted down to her level, put my hands on her eyes, and prayed a short prayer of healing in the name of Jesus. When I took my hands off of her eyes, I expected to see a happy little girl with good eyesight. She said that she could see well now, but she looked frightened.

Right after that her grandmother came up, and they started talking. The stout woman started motioning with her hands; she seemed overly excited. I found a translator who could explain to me what was going on. He told me why the little girl got so frightened. At the very moment I put my hands on her eyes, she saw a dark man, and then he left her. When she opened her eyes again, her eyesight was light and clear. The spirit of sickness had left her, but it was a frightening experience for the little girl.

Annelie Persson

# The Thick Glasses Were Now Unnecessary

In 2002, I went with Mission SOS to Bulgaria. The festival was held in a large sports arena, and every day thousands of people gathered to hear the message of Jesus Christ and have their needs met.

When the invitation for healing was made, people were streaming forward for us to pray for them. The first day of the festival I prayed with many people, but I didn't get to see any specific healing. Someone had pain in their back, another had pain in their leg, but it was hard to say if anyone had been healed. When I went back to where I was staying that evening, I was disappointed about this. Did I not have enough compassion and faith? Why didn't anything happen? I cried and prayed to God for forgiveness for my lack of love.

The next day during one of the most chaotic times of prayer for healing, when everyone was pulling and shoving for attention, a little seven-year-old girl came up to me. She wanted me to pray for her eyesight. I understood that immediately, since I noticed she wore such thick eyeglasses. I anointed her eyes with oil, and I remember praying, "OK, Lord, I can do absolutely nothing for this little girl to get back her eyesight. I pray in the name of Jesus that You will heal her." I took off her glasses and pulled out the SOS pamphlet "Saved in the Last Days," written in her language. She held it at normal distance and started to read. Her mother stood beside her and said that the little girl now could actually see and read the text! I was completely astonished and asked her to read more for me. She had received perfect eyesight! I was so happy and could not stop crying tears of joy and thankfulness to Jesus.

Lillemor Widell

# A Deaf and Mute Boy Was Healed

In February 2005, I was on a trip to Ghana with Mission SOS to be part of their "Signs and Wonders" festival in Bolgatanga, just a little south of the Sahara. Every evening after the sermon and the invitation for salvation, Johannes Amritzer asked for everyone who had sickness in their bodies to come forward for prayer. Many of the sick made their way forward; it was heartbreaking to see how many sicknesses and diseases these poor people had to live with.

I was standing in the middle of the sea of people and praying for the sick when a mother came forward with her six-year-old son. The boy, who in my eyes seemed to be completely well, had been deaf and mute since birth. He could not hear any sound from the speakers at the festival and had never been able to talk. I put my hands on him, and while I prayed, I felt in my spirit that there was a spirit of sickness in the little boy's head that closed his ears and bound his tongue. I commanded the spirit to leave in the name of Jesus, and immediately it was like someone had taken a hammer and hit the boy on the head! He suddenly was able to hear for the first time in his life—and the sound from the festival area was loud! The boy's eyes were big and wide, but he smiled from ear to ear and started to speak words that we were not able to understand! His mother cried and hugged her little boy as they went out from the crowded area and praised God as only Africans can!

Ari Mathisen

# Biblical Healing at a New Age Exhibit

This story is from an "inner harmony exhibit" in Stockholm. Approximately one million people in Sweden look to New Age to try to find the light, peace, harmony, power, and purpose for life that can be found only in Jesus Christ. They use crystals, methods of relaxation, the media, aura imaging, and lots of strange alternatives in order to seek a spiritual experience.

Thousands of people visit exhibitions where there are Reiki healers, fortune-tellers, and exorcists sharing a crowded space with representatives for expensive courses and salespeople for different kinds of natural products. Some of my friends and I thought that it would be suitable then to have a table for "the original source of power"—i.e., the Creator of Heaven and earth who loves these people! We used a language that New Age people understood, but without compromising an inch of the Gospel.

One day two teenage girls came by our table and looked at the sign that said: "Come and try the healing chair free! Biblical healing through the laying on of hands." The one girl used crutches and had suffered pain since she had twisted the bones in her leg and cracked her shins (shin splints). They wanted to know more.

"There is actually no magic in the chair itself," I said, "but inside of me lives Jesus in all His power. When I lay my hands on your leg, then there is transference of power."

That sounded good, they thought, so she laid her crutches aside and sat down in the chair.

"What shall I do while you are healing me?" the girl asked.

"Nothing. Just relax. I am going to pray and lay my hands on your leg. Many experience warmth or a shock like electricity when the power is transferred," I said.

So I laid my hands on her and prayed a simple prayer. I felt absolutely nothing myself, but during the whole time, she looked at me with very wide eyes. When I was finished, I asked her if she felt any difference.

"Yes! It felt really strange when you held your hand there. All the pain is gone! How in the world did you do that?"

She stood up and tested her weight on the leg, and then she stomped hard on the ground with her foot—she no longer felt any pain whatsoever!

Now both the girls were interested and hungry to know more. They had already tested New Age healing earlier, but it only worked a very short while, they said. This was something completely different. I showed them Isaiah 53, where Jesus took on Himself all our sicknesses. He totally wiped them out on the cross, but most of all, he took our shame and emptiness. When I had prayed for them once again, they went on their way. The girl was now holding the crutches in her hands.

Rickard Widell

# She Received Her Hearing Back

It was my first trip to Africa. The 2004 festival in Migori, Kenya, had already been going for several days, and Johannes Amritzer had preached and given an invitation for salvation. A woman came forward toward my friends and me when we were praying for people that needed healing. The woman had her daughter with her. Through sign and body language, we understood that the little girl was deaf in one ear.

We tested by snapping our fingers beside her ear; she did not react. My three Bible school friends and I anointed the little girl with oil and laid our hands on her ear. We commanded the deafness to go in the name of Jesus. When we had finished praying, we took our hands off her ear and checked her hearing. She still did not hear anything in the one ear. We then did the same thing again: we laid our hands on and around her ear and prayed for her. There was still no change.

After we had prayed three or four times for her, the last time quite angry at the deafness that would not loosen its grip, we asked a translator that walked by us to help us check her ear to see if she was healed. And she was! She could hear! The translator said some word in Swahili in her formerly deaf ear, while she covered the hearing ear; she repeated the word for us who were standing around. I will always carry this experience in my heart. It was the first "big healing" that God did through me; I saw that God could use even me.

Anna-Karin Carlsson

# Her Bones Moved!

Suddenly, she sat there in front of me on the lawn, right in front of the stage at the festival in Migori, Kenya, in 2004: a young woman around 20 years of age. Her right arm had been broken for more than six months and since then she had such excruciating pain that she could not move her arm at all. One could clearly see that one of the bones was completely broken off and pointing up toward the skin. The bone was approximately three to four centimeters in the wrong direction!

I heard the Holy Spirit whisper to me that I should speak to the bone that it should put itself into the right position again. Her arm started to shake violently. I asked her through the translator what had happened. With large tears in her eyes, the woman cried out: "I feel the bone moving!" When I looked down at her arm, I saw how the bone was shaking and moving itself into the right position. Full of the power of God, she unsteadily got up and raised her arm toward Heaven and waved it around in a circle several times! All the pain was gone! Jesus had really touched her, and it was wonderful to see her crying and laughing at the same time, standing and praising God with her arms raised high!

Lisa Pålsson

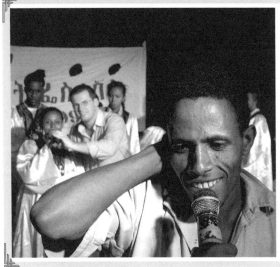

A twenty-five-year-old man was saved during the Signs & Wonders Festival in Dire Dawa, Ethiopia, in 2005.

That same night, God healed his deaf ear. With joy, his healing was established and proved through a hearing test on stage.

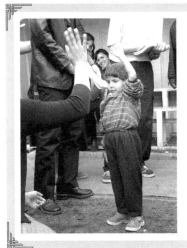

A five-year-old boy named Milcho had never been able to lift his left arm or move his left leg properly. He was completely healed after prayer in Pazardzik, Bulgaria, in 2002, and he proudly showed off his new skills.

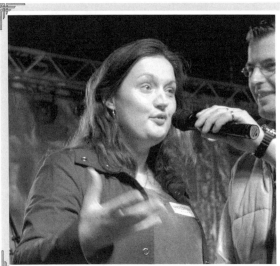

In the middle of Mission SOS's annual festival, Harvest Cry, Susann Hedman Niemi suddenly noticed how much easier it was to breathe.

She had suffered from exercise-induced asthma and asthma triggered by infection since the age of two. When she raced on stage to test her healing, she found that all her troubles were gone.

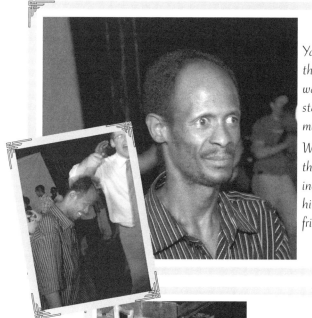

Yalow Haile was well-known in the Ethiopian city of Harar. He was working at the central gas station and had been deaf and mute since childhood.

When Jesus healed him in 2006, the festival area was filled with an incredible acclamation. Yalow himself was dancing with his friends. Jesus did a key miracle!

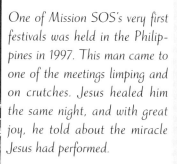

One of Mission SOS's very first festivals was held in the Philippines in 1997. This man came to one of the meetings limping and on crutches. Jesus healed him the same night, and with great joy, he told about the miracle Jesus had performed.

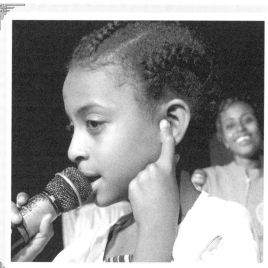

Matal Bagivond, nine years old, had been completely deaf in her right ear since birth.

When a team member from Mission SOS anointed her with oil and prayed for her during Mission SOS's festival in Dire Dawa, Ethiopia, in 2005, she was healed. After the healing, she could hear silent whispering and could repeat what she heard into the microphone.

This woman was a volunteer worker during the festival in the Bulgarian city of Pazardzik, in the spring of 2002. Her left eye was severely squinted; but after prayer, it twisted completely right.

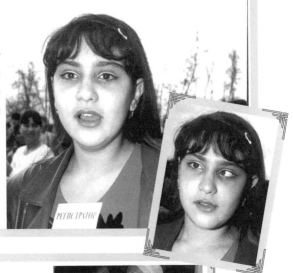

For sixteen years, this woman had been crawling on the city streets due to paralysis in her legs. During the last meeting of the festival in Bolgatanga, Ghana, in 2005, she was completely healed and could jump and dance on the stage before the crowd.

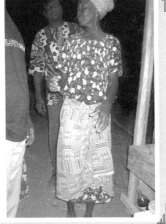

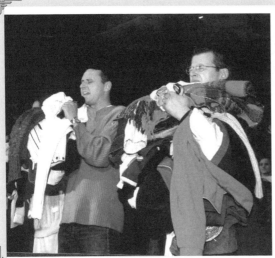

In a big tent meeting in the Swedish town of Nyhem, prayer cloths and clothes were brought to the stage for people to give to their sick friends and relatives who were at home.

A long time later, Mission SOS received several letters and phone calls regarding the testimonies of miracles that God had performed through the prayer cloths.

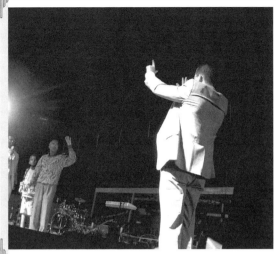

In Dire Dawa in 2005, this man had to be led by his son to the festival because of a severe vision defect.

The first night, he was healed by Jesus and has been able to see without any problems ever since. Here, his sight is being thoroughly tested.

When Mission SOS was in Dire Dawa in Ethiopia in 2005, one of the team members stepped in to a deaf school in the neighboring city of Harar.

Ten students of that school were healed and started to hear! Nine-year-old Hafiza Abdulkdr was one of the ten; here she is with her teacher.

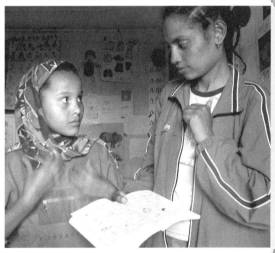

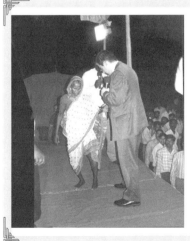

Shrija Slani was paralyzed on the left side of her body. When she listened to the preaching during the festival in Nagpur, India, in 2002, she received faith for a healing. All the attendants of the festival could see how she was completely healed and started to walk.

A deaf and mute boy in Pakistan was in total shock when he could hear himself babble and make sounds in the microphone! This happened in front of about 30,000 people during the festival in Karachi in 1999.

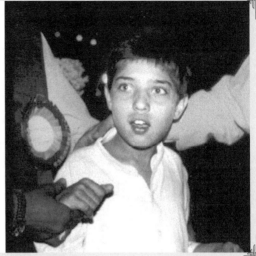

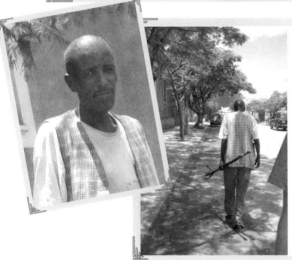

Luche Adam, forty-seven years old, was suffering from a broken left leg. He came with a crutch to a street meeting during the festival in Harar, Ethiopia, in 2006.

After the meeting and prayer, Luche walked away with the crutch in his hand, saved and healed!

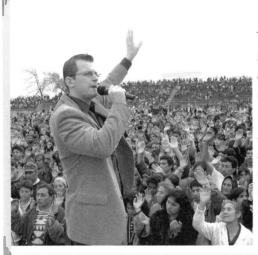

The soccer arena's home team had never attracted an audience as great as the audience that Jesus attracted in Pazardzik, Bulgaria, in 2002.

More than 5,500 people responded to the altar call during the five-day festival! Here we see hundreds of people giving their lives to Jesus.

# Other Books and Booklets by the Author

- *Baptized in Holy Spirit and Fire*
- *Practical Discipleship Training School*
- *Saved in the Last Days*
- *En ny missionsvåg (A New Missions Wave)*

For more information about
Johannes Amritzer and Mission SOS,
please visit
www.missionsos.com

Additional copies of this book and other book titles from DESTINY IMAGE™ EUROPE are available at your local bookstore.

We are adding new titles every month!

To view our complete catalog online, visit us at:
www.eurodestinyimage.com

Send a request for a catalog to:

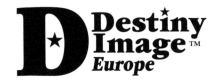

Via Acquacorrente, 6
65123 - Pescara - ITALY
Tel. +39 085 4716623 - Fax +39 085 9431270

*"Changing the world, one book at a time."*

---

Are you an author?

Do you have a "today" God-given message?

## CONTACT US

We will be happy to review your manuscript for a possible publishing:

publisher@eurodestinyimage.com